CARDIAC SURGERY
Current Issues 3

CARDIAC SURGERY
Current Issues   3

Edited by
Aurel C. Cernaianu
and
Anthony J. DelRossi

University of Medicine and Dentistry of New Jersey
Robert Wood Johnson Medical School at Camden
Camden, New Jersey

PLENUM PRESS • NEW YORK AND LONDON

Proceedings of the Fifth Annual Meeting on Cardiac Surgery: Current Issues, held
November 18–20, 1993, in St. Thomas, Virgin Islands

ISSN 1072-9798

ISBN 0-306-45015-1

© 1995 Plenum Press, New York
A Division of Plenum Publishing Corporation
233 Spring Street, New York, N. Y. 10013

10 9 8 7 6 5 4 3 2 1

All rights reserved

No part of this book may be reproduced, stored in a retrieval system, or transmitted in any
form or by any means, electronic, mechanical, photocopying, microfilming, recording, or
otherwise, without written permission from the Publisher

Printed in the United States of America

PREFACE

The topics in this book represent the presentations given at the Fifth Annual Meeting entitled "Cardiac Surgery: Current Issues" held at the Frenchman's Reef Beach Resort, St. Thomas, U.S. Virgin Islands, November 18-20, 1993.

This symposium was sponsored by the Division of Cardiothoracic Surgery, the School of Cardiovascular Perfusion and the Department of Nursing Education and Quality Assurance of Cooper Hospital/University Medical Center, the University of Medicine and Dentistry of New Jersey, Robert Wood Johnson Medical School, Camden, New Jersey, as well as the Academy of Medicine of New Jersey.

Chapter authors were charged with the task of writing brief overviews of major issues related to the field of cardiac surgery. The book is specifically tailored to the needs of cardiothoracic surgeons, cardiovascular perfusionists, allied health professionals and nursing personnel involved in all phases of caring for the cardiac surgical patient.

Although intended as a reference source with emphasis on up-dated approaches applied in cardiac surgery, it is hoped that the discussion of these topics will compliment other texts and manuscripts. Obviously, a book of this length cannot cover the whole multidisciplinary and complex field of cardiac surgery. However, co-editors are certain that the annual appearance of this text will highlight comprehensive, new and interesting approaches to the field of cardiac surgery.

The co-editors are greatly thankful to the contributors for their efforts in providing comprehensive chapters. Without their expertise, this work may not have been possible. We would also like to thank Ms. Eileen Bermingham and the staff at Plenum Publishing Corporation for their tremendous help in completing this work.

Aurel C. Cernaianu, M.D.
Anthony J. DelRossi, M.D.

CONTENTS

Mechanical Valves and the Small Aortic Annulus: Replacement
    Versus Root Enlargement 1
    Donald B. Doty, M.D.

Valve Repair in Acquired Heart Disease 7
    Robert B. Karp, M.D.

Valve Surgery Combined with Myocardial Revascularization 13
    Patrick M. McCarthy, M.D.

Failed PTCA: Myocardial Protection and Surgical Management in the
    Catheterization Laboratory 19
    Timothy J. Gardner, M.D.

Treatment of Acute Thoracic Aortic Dissections 27
    Jan D. Galla, M.D. and Randall B. Griepp, M.D.

Coarctation of the Aorta: Surgical Technique and Controversies 39
    Robert B. Karp, M.D.

Selection of Conduits for Primary and Re-Do Operations 45
    John L. Ochsner, M.D.

Surgical Treatment of Pediatric Aortic Stenosis 55
    Donald B. Doty, M.D.

Surgical and Bioengineering Advances in the Treatment of Life
    Threatening Ventricular Arrhythmias 65
    Alden H. Harken, M.D., Patricia A. Kelly, M.D.,
      David Mann, M.D., Roger S. Damle, M.D.,
      and Michael Reiter, M.D.

Less Heparin for Cardiopulmonary Bypass 77
    Ludwig K. von Segesser, M.D., Branko M. Weiss, M.D.,
      Michele Genoni, M.D., Boris Leskosek, and
      Marko I. Turina, M.D.

Blood Conservation in Cardiac Surgery 89
   John W. Hammon, Jr., M.D.

Patient Selection Criteria for Left Ventricular Assist
   Device Placement 99
   Mehmet C. Oz, M.D., Howard R. Levin, M.D.,
      Keith Reemtsma, M.D., and Eric A. Rose, M.D.

Support of the Failing Heart by Mechanical Devices 105
   William C. DeVries, M.D.

Ecmo in the 90's 135
   Sherry C. Faulkner, C.C.P.

Radiofrequency Ablation of Ventricular Tachycardia 143
   Joan M. Craney, R.N., M.S.N.

Update in Internal Cardioverter Defibrillators 149
   Julia Ann Purcell, R.N., M.N., C.C.R.N.

Hemodynamics in the Cardiothoracic Intensive Care Unit: The
   Nursing Prospective 157
   Mary Ellen Kern, R.N., M.S.N., C.C.R.N.

Thoracic Aortic Aneurysm Associated with Marfan Syndrome 165
   Jane V. Stewart, M.S.N., R.N., C.C.R.N.

Controversies in the Management of the Cardiac Surgical Patient 169
   Debra J. Lynn-McHale, M.S.N., R.N., C.C.R.N.

Rehabilitation Post Cardiac Surgery 175
   Susan G. Burrows, R.N., M.N.

Shifting Paradigms: Preparing Ourselves for the Next Century 183
   Jane C. Rothrock, D.N.Sc., R.N.

Contributors 187

Index 191

MECHANICAL VALVES AND THE SMALL AORTIC ANNULUS: REPLACEMENT VERSUS ROOT ENLARGEMENT

Donald B. Doty, M.D.

University of Utah School of Medicine
LDS Hospital
Salt Lake City, Utah

It is quite clear that all devices used to replace the aortic valve are at least mildly obstructive. When the aortic root is small the problem is worse. Choice of a replacement device for use in the small aortic root and the decision of whether or not to enlarge the outflow tract to accommodate a larger device are dilemmas which confront cardiac surgeons frequently.

ANATOMY OF THE AORTIC ROOT

Anderson and associates[1] have called attention to the fact that the word *annulus* when applied to the left ventricular outflow tract at the level of the aortic valve is a misnomer. *Annulus* defines a ring or circle and for surgeons the word suggests that there is a ring of fibrous connective tissue at the level of the aortic valve which can be measured and can be used to attach a prosthetic replacement device for the aortic valve. While such rings of fibrous tissue exist around the atrioventricular valves, there is absolutely no connective tissue ring which can be defined surrounding the semilunar valves. Surgeons are aware of this fact but the use of the word *annulus* persists perhaps because there is not a better term to describe the space of the left ventricular outflow tract at the level of the aortic valve or because surgeons are all used to the term and understand by inference what it means. Anderson prefers the term *ventriculoaortic junction* to describe a plane which is anatomically the junction made between the ventricle and the arterial trunk it supports. The aortic valve, with its semilunar shape has both, aortic and ventricular components across the ventriculoaortic junction. For the surgeon, this may produce some confusion because the plane which is generally understood as the *aortic annulus* is described best as the circular plane of the left ventricular outflow tract located at the lowest point of the fibrous attachment of the aortic valve leaflets (cusps) or the deepest point in the sinus of Valsalva. The diameter of the outflow tract at this plane is usually the narrow point in the left ventricular outflow tract (in pure valvular heart disease) and is used for determination of the diameter of the prosthetic device for valve replacement. It is possible that Anderson's slightly higher plane is a better description of where the prosthetic valve will actually be attached because the fibrous tissues at the depth of the sinus of Valsalva are probably pulled up to the sewing ring of the prosthesis and the tissues at the commissures are pulled down to some degree. In either case, it probably does not amount to much as a practical matter for the surgeon, who is mainly interested in identifying the diameter dimension at the level of the fibrous support of the aortic valve in order to choose an appropriate replacement prosthesis. An aortic annulus is considered small when the measured diameter is 21 mm or less. Anderson is right in suggesting that the term annulus be abandoned in favor of better understanding of normal and abnormal valvar morphology and function.

Anderson et al[1] describe the aortic root as the area of the left ventricular outflow tract supporting the leaflets of the aortic valve taking the form of a cylinder in which the three leaflets are attached by fibrous tissue in the fashion of three half-moons. The fibrous attachments rise to an apex or touching point defined as the commissure. The triangular space formed beneath the apices of the fibrous commissures is called the interleaflet triangle. There is no fibrous connective tissue in the interleaflet triangle but rather there is only a thin layer of the arterial wall separating the inside of the left ventricle from the extracardiac space. These triangles are differentiated from the fibrous trigones (right and left) which represent the two ends of the fibrous continuity of the anterior leaflet of the mitral valve and the aortic valve. The fibrous trigones are part of the fibrous skeleton on the heart. McAlpin[2] has shown that the commissure between the left and non-coronary sinuses is positioned directly above the mid-point of the anterior leaflet of the mitral valve. This anatomic landmark is important in operations designed to enlarge the aortic root posteriorly. The interleaflet triangle beneath this posterior commissure is composed of a quite loose and pliable tissue which is positioned above the hinge point of the anterior leaflet of the mitral valve. Incision into these tissues allows the aortic root to be opened and enlarged by separation of these tissues without incision of the anterior leaflet of the mitral valve or opening the left atrium.

Ross[3] has pointed out that preoccupation with the concept of an aortic *ring* gave rise to mechanical and bioprosthetic aortic replacement devices based on a ring or single-suture-line replacement technique. All these devices are based on mechanisms which result in turbulent blood flow which cause energy loss across the valve and cause obstructive pressure gradients. This explains why aortic allografts are the least obstructive of all devices used for replacement of the aortic valve.[4]

CHOICE OF REPLACEMENT DEVICE FOR THE AORTIC VALVE IN THE SMALL AORTIC ROOT

All devices used to replace the aortic valve with small annulus are mildly stenotic.[4] Aortic allografts are the least obstructive followed by the

St. Jude Medical prosthesis (St. Jude Medical, Inc., St. Paul, Minnesota). Porcine heterografts are not as good hemodynamically in the small aortic root. The real question is what is the smallest size of a prosthesis tolerated in the aortic root which will achieve valve function without producing obstruction which may affect long-term function of the left ventricle. There should be a size limit which is related to flow across the valve. Achieving maximal flow (cardiac output) during exercise and measuring pressure gradient across the prosthesis should provide the information which sets the limit for the lowest tolerable size (diameter) of a prosthetic valve. There have only been a few attempts by investigators to establish these limits by exercise testing and there are no clear established guidelines.[5] Surgeons have set their own limits for what is tolerable in terms of prosthetic size based on very sparse information and documentation. It is of considerable interest that body surface area (BSA) is better related to pressure gradient than flow or cardiac output.[4] Perhaps this is an explanation for why some patients will tolerate a 21 mm prosthesis and others will show high resting and exercise pressure gradients across the prosthesis. Non-invasive postoperative doppler echocardiography has provided estimation of pressure gradients across small aortic prostheses during rest and exercise.[6] There are apparently some technical considerations when using doppler ultrasound for calculating pressure gradients across mechanical prosthetic heart valves due to artifact created by turbulent flow.[7] Nevertheless, these data are presently the only useful information to determine hemodynamics during rest and exercise aside from transatrial septal cardiac catheterization. Prohibitive pressure gradients are observed during exercise in patients having 19 mm prostheses. Patients with 21 mm prostheses will demonstrate higher gradients especially during exercise. Some of the measured values are above 30 mm Hg which is much higher than those in patients having 23 mm prostheses, however statistical difference could be demonstrated. It has been concluded from these data that the break point for acceptable prosthetic valve diameter for adult patients requiring aortic valve replacement is 21 mm. Prosthetic valve diameter of 23 mm or greater are acceptable especially when modern mechanical devices are used. The insertion of a 21 mm diameter prosthesis requires some judgement related to the patient's body size and anticipated level of activity. Prosthetic valve diameter 19 mm and below should be avoided. The most significant paper to dispute this principle[8] is seriously flawed because the parameters used to measure success (raw survival and functional class) are too gross and neglect the potential for long-term detrimental effects of ventricular hypertrophy resulting from chronic left ventricular outflow obstruction by a prosthesis which is too small for the patient. The data plots presented in this paper show wide scatter with many individual patients showing resting pressure gradients exceeding 30 mm Hg at rest. It is interesting that BSA was not correlated to high resting pressure gradient in 35 percent (6 of 17) of patients having BSA less than 1.5 m^2 and resting pressure gradient greater than 30 mm Hg. Actuarial survival was 71 percent at ten years following implantation of a 17 or 19 mm aortic valve prosthesis but the authors discounted these data on the basis that associated coronary artery disease was not uniformly treated.

The issue of prosthetic valve size has been further clouded by the contention that the manufacturer's stated diameter of the prosthesis may not actually correlate with the tissue annulus diameter into which the prosthesis may be accommodated.[9] For example, one manufacturer's modified 20 mm valve will fit into the same diameter which may only accommodate another manufacturer's 19 mm valve. Thus, we observe the current trend to decrease the size of sewing ring of small aortic prostheses to fit a larger mechanical device into a smaller space, in order to gain more flow area. A recent study[10] of 20 mm Medtronic-Hall (Medtronic, Inc., Minneapolis, Minnesota) versus 19 mm St. Jude medical aortic prostheses using doppler ultrasound and dobutamine induced increased cardiac output showed no difference between these valves at rest in terms of gradient or effective flow area. However, the Medtronic-Hall pivoting disk valve required lesser driving pressure to generate similar flows. One wonders what would have been the result of such study if truly size-matched mechanical devices had been compared.

It is concluded that 19 mm aortic prostheses should not be used for replacement of the aortic valve in any adult. The 21 mm prosthesis and even an occasional 23 mm prosthesis may develop significant pressure gradients during exercise. The place of modified mechanical valves with reduced sewing rings has yet to be determined. These 19, 20 and 21 mm size valves may be useful as long as the surgeon understands clearly the specifications of the device that is actually being implanted relative to data which is known on standard prostheses. A safe policy is not to implant an aortic valve prosthesis smaller than 23 mm unless the patient is sedentary and has a BSA less than 1.5 m^2. In these unusual circumstances, a 21 mm mechanical prosthesis may be adequate.

ENLARGEMENT OF THE AORTIC ROOT

There is temptation to force an oversized aortic prosthesis into the aortic root in hopes of gaining better hemodynamic performance. Every surgeon who has tried to do this, has been faced with the consequences of having difficulty to close the aortotomy over the large prosthetic device and the horrible prospective of bleeding which may accompany insecure or inadequate aortic closure. Should the surgeon think there may be difficult closing of the aorta, a patch may be easily inserted to achieve aortic closure without tension. Oversize prostheses may also erode the fibrous structure of the aortic root making subsequent operation more difficult should this be required. Forcing in an oversized prosthesis should be avoided. It is better to enlarge the aortic root primarily to accommodate a proper size prostheses.

The aortic root may be enlarged sufficiently by a posterior patch in most instances. An anterior enlargement by aortoventriculoplasty (Konno-Rastan procedure)[11] is only required in children or in complex left ventricular outflow obstruction with a significant sub-valvular obstructive component. Posterior enlargement of the aortic root is accomplished by extending the aortotomy through the fibrous structure of the aortic valve to allow separation of the tissues sufficiently to accommodate a patch to enlarge the circumference of the aortic root. The incision may be extended into the anterior leaflet of the mitral valve to allow even greater separation of the tissues and incorporation of a larger patch. Nicks et al[12] described an extension of the aortotomy with incision of the fibrous support of the aortic valve in the non-coronary sinus into the anterior leaflet of the mitral valve. Others have described modifications of the posterior aortic root enlargement technique. The most anatomic approach has been presented by Manougian et al.[13] and of Nunez et al.[14] The incision of the fibrous structure of the aortic valve is made through the commissure joining the non-coronary and the left coronary cusps. The incision includes the loose tissues of the interleaflet triangle. Sufficient separation of the tissues can often be obtained without incising the anterior leaflet of the mitral valve. Should greater enlargement be desired, the incision in the mitral valve will be exactly at the mid-point of the anterior leaflet. Reconstruction of the mitral valve should be more anatomic and reliable.

Posterior root enlargement procedures are easy to perform and are not associated with increase in operative morbidity or mortality.[15] Approximately 45 minutes are added to the operation to perform the root enlargement.[13] Enlargement of the aortic root to accommodate a prosthesis with hemodynamically better performance is superior to implanting a prosthesis which is too small.

REFERENCES

1. Anderson RH, Devine WA, Ho SY, Smith A, McKay R: The myth of the aortic annulus: the anatomy of the subaortic outflow tract. Ann Thorac Surg 1991;52:640–46.
2. McAlpin WA: Heart and Coronary Arteries. Springer-Verlag, New York, NY, 1975:10.
3. Ross DN: Editorial: Left ventricular outflow tract: Some lessons learned. J Heart Valve Dis 1993;2:63–65.
4. Jaffe WM, Coverdale A, Roche AHG, Whitlock RML, Neutze JM, Barratt-Boyes BG: Rest and exercise hemodynamics of 20 to 23 mm allograft, Medtronic Intact (porcine), and St. Jude Medical valves in the aortic position. J Thorac Cardiovasc Surg 1990;100:167–174.
5. Kirklin JW, Barratt-Boyes BG: Cardiac Surgery 2 Ed. Churchill Livingstone, New York, NY, 1993:539.
6. Teoh KH, Fulop JC, Weisel RD, Ivanov J, Tong CP, Slattery SA, Radowski H: Aortic valve replacement with a small prosthesis. Circulation 1987;76(suppl III):123–130.
7. Wiseth R, Levang OW, Sande E, Tangen G, Skjaerpe T, Hatle L: Hemodynamic evaluation by doppler echocardiography of small prostheses and bioprostheses in the aortic valve position. Amer J Cardiol 1992;70:240–46.
8. Foster AH, Tracy CM, Greenberg GJ, McIntosh CL, Clark RE: Valve replacement in narrow aortic roots: serial hemodynamics and long-term clinical outcome. Ann Thorac Surg 1986;42:506–516.
9. Bonchek LI, Burlingame MW, Vaazales BE: Accuracy of sizers for aortic valve prostheses. J Thorac Cardiovasc Surg 1987;94:632–34.
10. Bednarz J, Marcus R, Lupovitch S, Piccione W, Abruzzo J, Vandenberg B, Mulhern K, Borok R, Kerber RE, Lang R: Dobutamine-induced flow augmentation for assessment of small diameter aortic prostheses: Comparative study of bileaflet and pivoting disc valves. Circulation 1993;88:I-539.
11. Doty DB: Cardiac Surgery - A Looseleaf Workbook and Update Service. Chicago, Year Book Medical Publishers, 1985; chp LVOTO.
12. Nicks R, Cartmill T, Bernstein L: Hypoplasia of the aortic root: the problem of aortic valve replacement. Thorax 1970;25:339–46.
13. Manouguian S, Seybold-Epting W: Patch enlargement of the aortic valve ring by extending the aortic incision into the anterior mitral leaflet. J Thorac Cardiovasc Surg 1979;78:402–412.
14. Nunez L, Aguado MG, Pinto AG, Larrea JL: Enlargement of the aortic annulus by resecting the commissure between the left and non-coronary cusps. Texas Heart Inst J 1983;10:301–303.

15. Pugliese P, Bernabei M, Santi C, Pasque A, Eufrate S: Posterior enlargement of the small annulus during aortic valve replacement versus implantation of a small prosthesis. Ann Thorac Surg 1984;38:31–36.

VALVE REPAIR IN ACQUIRED HEART DISEASE

Robert B. Karp, M.D.

The University of Chicago
Pritzker School of Medicine
Chicago, Illinois

Because there are some relative disadvantages of all cardiac valve replacement devices, there is a continuing interest in repair of diseased valves, rather than replacement. Most of the focus of any discussion of valve repair resides at the atrioventricular valve level, particularly the mitral valve. However, there is some interest in repair of the aortic valve. For example, Duran[1], Carpentier[2], and Cosgrove et al.[3] each have reported small series of suture annuloplasty of the aortic ring to diminish or control aortic incompetence. Basically, an encircling purse-string suture is placed at the base of the aortic cusps and tightened such as to narrow the ventricular aortic junction. Occasionally, a triangular resection of redundant cusp tissue is used. David and Filindel[4] have described the preservation of the native aortic valve in annular dilatation by scalloping the aortic sinuses and encasing the aortic valve complex in a Dacron tube, and subsequent reattachment of the coronary ostia.

Recently, debridement of diseased valves with pure aortic stenosis has resurfaced. We have a small group of 15 patients in whom ultrasonic surgical debridement has been satisfactorily accomplished.[5] Using the CUSA aspirating vibrating debriding device (Valley Labs, Boulder, CO), operating loops, and additional suction and irrigation, meticulous debridement of the aortic cusps can be accomplished. Candidates for this technique are not frequent. Our usual indications are those patients having concomitant coronary artery bypass grafting in whom there is moderate, degenerative aortic stenosis, no aortic incompetence, and no fusion of the valve commissures. The CUSA device is applied until the valve cusps are made pliable and can be made to easily fold back into and conform to the sinuses of Valsalva. We have had one early and one late failure in this group. The average mean gradients have decreased from approximately 40 mm Hg to 9 mm Hg when measured early postoperatively by echocardiography. In contrast to some other series, the incidence of aortic incompetence has been quite low, with only one thromboembolic event. The operation requires no anticoagulation and, of course, the native aortic valve is preserved.

The remainder of this discussion is devoted to mitral valve repair. In 1985, Sand et al.[6] reviewed the collective experience with mitral valve repair between 1967 and 1983 at the University of Alabama. Reparative techniques varied from simple and perhaps primitive early commissural annuloplasty techniques to those more sophisticated techniques later expounded by Carpentier and others. We found that patients having mitral valve repair (n=131) had significantly better long-term survival than a large separate group of patients undergoing replacement. For instance, actuarial survival of those having valve replacement in all functional categories was 60 percent at five years. Actuarial survival of those having repair at five years was 80 percent ($p=.005$). Admittedly, the severity indexes of the two groups cannot be comparable. Similarly, a report by Colvin and Spencer[7] from New York University covering about the same time period showed a superiority in survival with patients having mitral valve repair compared to those having replacement either with a mechanical or tissue valve.

The report of Sand et al. was particularly encouraging when the patients having valve repair were compared to those having valve replacement in terms of re-operation. There was a slight superiority and freedom from re-operation in those having repair versus those having valve replacement. Approximately 93 percent of those having repair were free of re-operation at five years. Additionally, there seemed to be no increasing late incidence of re-operation in the repair group.

The mitral valve apparatus is a complex arrangement of two leaflets, with primary, secondary, and tertiary supporting chords, and two papillary muscles. In turn, the papillary muscle position and function is largely determined by the geometry and function of the left ventricle. The anterior leaflet of the mitral valve is a large, trapezoidal structure with a rather narrow and limited insertion bordering on the left ventricular outflow tract. It is separated from the narrower and more broadly based posterior leaflet by the anterolateral and posterior medial commissures. When viewed by the surgeon through a lateral opening into the left atrium, the circumference of the base of the mitral leaflets (so called mitral annulus) is related in clockwise fashion to the atrioventricular node, the posterior medial commissure, the coronary sinus, the atrioventricular nodal artery, the circumflex coronary artery, the anterolateral commissure, the aortic root, and finally the central fibrous body. Potentially, any of these structures is at risk when suturing in the mitral valve area.

One cannot have any acquaintance at all with techniques and advantages of mitral valve repair without having read the work of Carpentier and colleagues[2] from Paris, France. These investigators have classified mitral valve disease in terms of pathophysiology, i.e., restrictive, dilated, or degenerative, and in terms of anatomy. Moreover, they have introduced concepts for valve repair directed at the relieving commissural fusion and subcommisural fusion. Their techniques have been focussed particularly at repairing chordal rupture, leaflet prolapse, and annular dilatation.

Perhaps the most frequent reparative operation for mitral incompetence is that involving a quadrangular resection of a portion of the posterior leaflet. The repair of that defect is performed with interrupted sutures and narrowing and buttressing of the annulus with a supportive ring. Important concepts to this type of operation are the fact that the anterior leaflet has a fixed and rather narrow base while the posterior leaflet has a longer circumferential base and therefore, the latter may be narrowed by a purse-string or ring annuloplasty. For specific areas of prolapse on the anterior leaflet, a triangular resection is usually less extensive than when the quadrangular resection is performed. Often, this is accompanied by chordal transfer or insertion of Goretex suture to perform the function of an artificial chordae tendineae. Both anterior and posterior resections are almost universally accompanied by a supportive ring to remodel and narrow the often dilated annulus. The Carpentier-Edwards® ring is semi-rigid. Others have suggested that mitral valve function is less disturbed using a more flexible ring of either Dacron or bolstered pericardium. The ring is placed such that the tissue of the insertion of the posterior leaflet which occupies about two-thirds of the mitral annulus is gathered and purse-stringed to narrow the annulus posteriorly. Complimentary mitral annuloplastic techniques also include chordal shortening and chordal transfer. In the shortening procedure, the offending elongated chorda is doubled upon itself and inverted into its origin at the papillary muscle. Chordal transfer involves generally moving a portion of the attachment of a posterior medial chorda tendineae anteriorly to support a prolapsing anterior leaflet. The defect in the posterior leaflet is closed in a quadrangular way, and the repair is bolstered with a Carpentier-Edwards® ring.

The obvious advantage of mitral repair over mitral replacement lies in the non-use of a prosthetic device and the lack of the attendant prosthetic complications such as anticoagulation, thromboembolism, thrombosis, and prosthetic valve infection. Recently, it has been generally acknowledged that mitral valve repair by retaining the support and tension mechanism of the mitral valve and by retaining more or less the geometry of the left ventricle, may result in better ventricular contractility as compared to resection of the mitral apparatus. It is well know that mitral valve operation, particularly replacement, in the setting of chronic mitral regurgitation often results in a decrement of contractility indices postoperatively. This may be due to a change in ventricular geometry, a lack of tensor apparatus, or particularly, the elimination of a low impedance resistor, (the left atrium), during left ventricular systolic ejection. In mitral incompetence, there is no isovolemic ventricular contraction. Thus, with restoration of mitral competence, load resisting left ventricular shortening is increased, oxygen demand increases, and ejection fraction has been shown to decrease. Both clinically and experimentally, retention of the mitral tensor apparatus has resulted in better contractile indices in mitral valve surgery. For instance, Tirone David has evidence in operative patients postoperatively after repair have better ejection fractions than after replacement. In elegant studies from Stanford, Miller and his colleagues[8] have demonstrated in experimental animals that precise indices of contractility such as pressure volume curves and elastance are directly related to *in-vitro* measurements with intact then detached then reattached chordae tendineae. The detached chorda tendineae having less good contractile indices.

In a brief review of our own recent experience, we looked at 6 patients having repair for either stenosis, insufficiency, or the combined lesion. There were six deaths. In 17 patients with mitral stenosis, there was no mortality. In 47 patients operated upon for mitral incompetence, there were six deaths, and in the combined lesion in two patients there were no deaths. Of importance was the etiologic grouping of these patients. There were no deaths in 25 patients with rheumatic disease, and in 12 patients with degenerative disease. On the contrary, in 13 patients with ischemic mitral incompetence, there were four deaths, and in 10 patients excluding the infant and neonatal group, there were no deaths in those with congenital mitral incompetence. If the mitral valve repair was performed as an isolated procedure, there were no deaths is 34 patients. When coronary artery bypass grafting was performed in conjunction with the mitral valve repair, there were four deaths in 18 patients. If other procedures were done, there were two deaths in 14 patients. The average age of the survivors was 50.4 years, the average age of the non-survivors was 70.2 years. It has become apparent to us, both from our own experience and that of others, that the primary determinant for survival in repair or replacement for mitral incompetence is ischemic heart disease. If the mitral incompetence is the result of an ischemic cardiomyopathy or an acute myocardial infarction, the mortality varies between 10 and 20 percent. For instance, in 39 patients having either repair or replacement of the mitral valve in severe incompetence associated with ischemic heart disease, there were eight deaths (20.5 percent). In 33 patients having either repair or replacement for mitral incompetence without ischemic disease, there were two deaths (6.1 percent).

In the 60 survivors with mitral valve repair, 35 were evaluated within the first year after the reparative procedure by transthoracic echocardiogram. Twenty-four revealed either no or trivial leakage, ten had mild leakage, and only one had moderate to severe leakage. That single individual with moderate leakage ultimately had a re-operation and mitral valve replacement.

In order to adequately perform mitral valve repair, one must have a in-depth knowledge of the normal anatomy of the valvular apparatus. One must be able to evaluate the valve precisely, using techniques to elongate and stretch the chordae, to recognize the commissures, and particularly to identify deviations from the horizontal plane of the mitral valve orifice. One must recognize scarring of the leaflets and of the papillary muscles, and promptly identify shortening of leaflets and or chordae. Certainly, the most obvious finding in degenerative mitral incompetence is a tear of one or two chordae tendineae. Additionally in our practice, we always assume that annular dilatation is present and therefore generally apply annuloplastic methods, either a variation of the Reed measured posterior annuloplasty or more frequently, the use of remodeling annuloplasty rings. In general, we apply several techniques using an eclectic approach; triangular and quadrangular resection when appropriate, chordal shortening, chordal transfer, and artificial Goretex chorda tendinea.

Using an assiduous diagnostic approach intraoperatively and eclectic annuloplastic methods, we have found that an aggressive approach to mitral valve repair is rewarded by satisfactory survival figures, and maintenance of mitral valve competence.

REFERENCES

1. Duran CG: Reconstructive techniques for rheumatic aortic valve disease. J Card Surg 1988;3:23–28.
2. Carpentier A: Cardiac valve surgery: the French correction. J Thor Cardiovasc Surg 1983;86:323–337.
3. Cosgrove DM, Ratliff NB, Schoff HV, Edwards WD: Aortic valve decalcification history repeated with a new result. Ann Thorac Surg 1990;49:689–690.
4. David TE, Filindel CM: An aortic valve repairing operation for patients with aortic incompetence and aneurysm of the ascending aorta. J Thor Cardiovasc Surg 1992;103:617–622.
5. Scott WJ, Neumann AL, Karp RB: Ultrasonic debridement of the aortic valve with 6-month echocardiographic followup. Am J Cardiol 1989;64:1206–1209.
6. Sand ME, Naftel DC, Blackstone EH, Kirklin JW, Karp RB: A comparison of repair and replacement for mitral valve incompetence. J Thorac Cardiovasc Surg 1987;94:208–219.
7. Spencer FC, Colvin SB, Culliford AT, Isom OW: Experiences with the Carpentier technique of mitral valve reconstruction in 103 patients (1980–1985). J Thorac Cardiovasc Surg 1985; Sup90(3):341–50.
8. Sarris GE, Cahill PD, Hansen DE, et al: Restoration of left ventricular systolic performance after reattachment of the mitral chordae tendineae. The importance of valvular-ventricular interaction. J Thorac Cardiovasc Surg 1988;95:969–979.

VALVE SURGERY COMBINED WITH MYOCARDIAL REVASCULARIZATION

Patrick M. McCarthy, M.D.

Cleveland Clinic Foundation
Cleveland, Ohio

The association of valve disease with coronary artery disease is frequently encountered in clinical cardiac surgery. Approximately one-third of the patients undergoing valve surgery at the Cleveland Clinic in recent years have also had concomitant coronary artery bypass (Figure 1).

In addition, it is well-recognized that the operative mortality for patients undergoing combined valve and coronary bypass surgery is significantly higher than for either valve surgery alone, or coronary bypass alone (Figure 2). It is also accepted that the operative mortality for valve repair is generally lower than for valve replacement.[1] Because of the increased

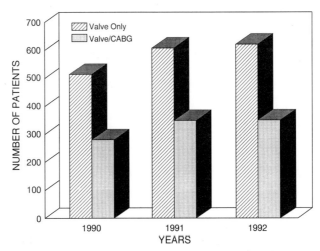

Figure 1. Approximately one-third of valve operations include concomitant coronary artery bypass. For example, in 1992, 634 patients underwent isolated valve surgery at the Cleveland Clinic, and 335 patients (34.6 percent of all valve operations) had combined valve/CABG.

Cardiac Surgery: Current Issues 3, Edited by A. C. Cernaianu and A. J. DelRossi,
Plenum Press, New York, 1995

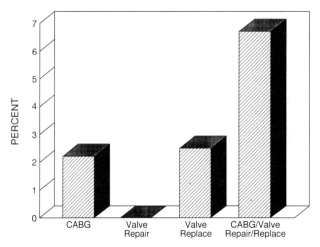

Figure 2. The in-hospital mortality for combined valve/CABG is higher than for either valve only or CABG only. In general, the mortality is lower for isolated valve repair (0 percent in 1992, n=149) than for valve replacement.

operative risk, it is appropriate that the surgeon have a clear understanding and approach to patients with combined valve and coronary lesions.

Several decisions are important when facing a patient with the possible combination of valve disease and coronary disease. First, in regard to the valve, the surgeon needs an excellent assessment of the degree of valve pathology, and the mechanism of valve pathology. Second, the surgeon must decide regarding valve repair versus valve replacement. This is an individual decision based upon the surgeon's experience, the mechanism of valve pathology, and the perceived risks and benefits for the individual patient. Finally, if the decision is made to replace the valve, a variety of valve types are available from which to choose. In regard to the associated coronary artery disease, the decision needs to be made whether or not there is an indication to perform coronary angiogram before anticipated valve surgery. If significant coronary disease is identified (greater than 50 percent stenosis), the choice of conduit for bypass grafting has to be decided. Finally, important decisions are made intraoperatively regarding the optimum myocardial protection. This brief chapter will review our general approach to these patients at the Cleveland Clinic. Of course, considerable flexibility is necessary with this diverse patient group.

PREOPERATIVE CONSIDERATIONS

For patients who are undergoing valve surgery *guidelines* to perform coronary angiography are appropriate. In general, coronary angiography is performed routinely for patients over the age of 40 years. Coronary angiograms are obtained selectively in patients less than 40 years of age who have a positive stress test, strong family history of coronary disease, or other risk factors (e.g. smoking, diabetes, high cholesterol). Coronary angiograms are generally avoided for patients with aortic valve endocarditis because of the risk of embolizing vegetations while manipulating catheters into the coronary ostia.

The cardiac valves are carefully assessed in patients undergoing coronary artery bypass. A history of rheumatic fever, or physical findings of valve disease, will prompt echocardiographic examination. Routine left ventriculography during left heart catheterization also may identify valve lesions. For patients with mild to moderate mitral valve lesions, we frequently plan for intraoperative transesophageal echocardiography to make the final decision regarding the need for valve surgery.

The decision regarding valve replacement for an individual patient is sometimes difficult and needs to be discussed with the patient before surgery. In general, for mechanical valve replacement (patients less than 65 years of age without significant bleeding disorder, and older patients with chronic atrial fibrillation) then we favor a St. Jude valve (St. Jude Medical, Inc., St. Paul, Minnesota). For patients in whom we use a bioprosthetic valve (e.g. greater than 65 years of age, contraindications to anticoagulation), we have favored the use of the Carpentier-Edwards mitral valve prosthesis (Baxter Healthcare Corp., Edwards CVS Division, Irvine, CA); and more recently, the Baxter-Edwards pericardial valve for use in the aortic position. In our experience (manuscript in progress) with 310 patients from 1982 to 1985, the Carpentier-Edwards pericardial bioprosthesis was free of structural valve deterioration at 10 years in 95 percent of patients over 65 years of age.[2]

INTRAOPERATIVE CONSIDERATIONS

Transesophageal echocardiography is used routinely during valve operations at the Cleveland Clinic in whom the possibility of valve repair is anticipated.[3] Pre-repair assessment of the underlying mechanism of valvular insufficiency, and the extent of pathology helps guide the surgeon. In addition, echocardiographic findings such as severe subvalvular disease and calcification in a patient with rheumatic valve disease may predispose the surgeon towards valve replacement rather than valve repair. Milder degrees of mitral regurgitation (e.g. 2+ on a scale to 4) may become more significant by transiently raising the arterial pressure (afterload) with phenylephrine hydrochloride. We routinely add mitral valve repair to coronary artery bypass patients with greater than or equal to 3+ mitral regurgitation, and selectively for patients with 2+ regurgitation with structural valve problems (e.g. leaflet prolapse).

Myocardial protection can be challenging because of the frequent coexistence of myocardial hypertrophy and multiple coronary blockages. We use combined antegrade and retrograde cardioplegia for this patient population. In particular, retrograde cardioplegia simplifies the valve portion of the operation because the *flow* of the operation does not have to be interrupted to administer cardioplegia. To better maintain protection of the right ventricle, we also use cardioplegia through the right coronary vein grafts.

The choice of conduit for coronary bypass is sometimes difficult. Although we use the internal mammary artery in the vast majority of patients,[4] and both internal mammary arteries frequently,[5] this strategy is not always appropriate. In particular, we do not use the internal mammary artery to replace patent vein bypass grafts at reoperations.[6] We may not choose to use it in older patients with severe left ventricular hypertrophy (e.g. aortic stenosis) and only a moderate (50 percent obstruction) left anterior descending stenosis. A saphenous vein graft may supply more flow in this instance, with less risk for competitive flow. In general, however, use of the internal mammary artery is very safe, even in the setting of reoperations.[7]

SPECIFIC VALVE/CORONARY BYPASS COMBINATIONS

Mitral regurgitation is sometimes associated with coronary artery disease, because of a causal relationship. Myocardial infarction can precipitate mitral regurgitation either acutely (e.g., papillary muscle rupture), or chronically with infarction and lengthening of the papillary muscle. Also, patients with ischemic cardiomyopathy and severe ventricular dysfunction and dilatation show a typical pattern of mitral regurgitation. The dilated ventricle leads to papillary muscle displacement, restricted leaflet motion and poor coaptation, annular dilatation, and a central jet of mitral regurgitation seen on echocardiogram.[3] With infarction or rupture of a papillary muscle, the jet of mitral regurgitation is usually eccentric.

A recent study from the Cleveland Clinic reviewed our experience with mitral valve repair for ischemic disease.[8] Eighty-four patients underwent mitral valve procedures for ischemic mitral regurgitation from 1985 until 1989 (6.5 percent of the 1,292 mitral valve operations during that same time). In 65 patients (77 percent), mitral valve repair was performed with coronary bypass, due to favorable anatomy and the preference of the operating surgeon. The mean age of these 65 patients was 66±10 years. They were New York Heart functional class 3.2±0.7 before surgery, and 53.8 percent of the patients were female.

Eighty-five percent of the patients (n=54) presented with chronic mitral pathology; and in 17 percent (n=11), it was an acute problem, five of these patients were in shock. The pathology was further divided into two groups, 39 patients with restricted valve leaflet function secondary to ventricular dilatation and ischemic cardiomyopathy (60 percent) and those with prolapse of the valve leaflet from either papillary muscle rupture (8 patients) or papillary muscle infarction (18 patients). Ventricular function was moderately or severely impaired in 65 percent of patients and was worse in the patients with restricted pathology.

Overall operative mortality was 9.2 percent and was not significantly different whether the pathology was prolapsed or restricted valve leaflet, or the pathology was of acute or chronic onset. However, long-term survival was markedly diminished in the restricted valve leaflet group secondary to the underlying ischemic cardiomyopathy (Figure 3). From this study, we concluded that mitral repair for ischemic disease is an uncommon cause of mitral valve surgery. Both acute and chronic causes are amenable to repair. A low operative mortality is obtainable with both, however, long-term survival is superior for those patients who have prolapse of the valve leaflets.

An earlier study from the Cleveland Clinic reviewed 300 patients with mitral valve *replacement* and coronary bypass from 1970 to 1983.[9] Ischemic

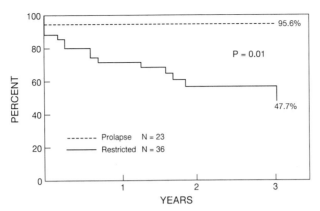

Figure 3. Long-term survival for patients with ischemic mitral regurgitation secondary to valve prolapse is good. Decreased survival for patients with restrictive leaflet motion (ischemic cardiomyopathy) relates to the underlying poor ventricular function. (Reproduced with permission from Hendren, et al; Ann Thorac Surg 1991;52:1246-52).

mitral regurgitation was the cause for surgery in 47 patients. The majority of patients had myxoid degeneration (147 patients) or rheumatic valve disease (102 patients). Operative mortality varied depending upon the underlying etiology. For those patients with myxoid valve disease, the operative mortality was 5.4 percent, for those with the combination of rheumatic valve disease and coronary disease, it was 8.8 percent, and for those with ischemic mitral regurgitation requiring valve replacement, it was 10.6 percent. Multivariate analysis identified radiographic cardiac enlargement, preoperative paced rhythm or atrial fibrillation, 70 percent or greater left main coronary obstruction, and serum bilirubin greater than 2 mg/dL as factors associated with in-hospital mortality. Risk factors for decreasing long-term survival included in-hospital ventricular arrhythmias, left ventricular dysfunction, and rheumatic or ischemic causes of mitral valve disease. Also, patients with bioprostheses without warfarin anticoagulation had better survival and event-free survival than those with bioprostheses taking warfarin and those with mechanical prostheses with or without warfarin.

The combination of aortic stenosis and coronary artery disease are particularly dangerous and can lead to severe myocardial ischemia. Adding coronary artery bypass to aortic valve replacement can increase operative mortality. Also, most patients with combined aortic stenosis and coronary artery disease are elderly, and frequently have comorbid conditions.

In 1988, we reported 375 patients who underwent aortic valve replacement for aortic stenosis with coronary bypass from 1981 until 1986.[10] The mean number of grafts per patient was 2.1. Moderate or severe ventricular dysfunction was present in 35 percent and 35 percent were greater or equal to 70 years of age. The in-hospital mortality was 5.3 percent. By multivariate analysis, Lytle found that the most significant risks for operative mortality ($p=0.008$) were female gender (3.9 percent mortality for males vs. 11.4 percent for females). Left ventricular dysfunction was also a significant predictor ($p=0.002$) of mortality (2.5 percent for patients with normal or mild ventricular dysfunction vs. 10.3 percent for patients with moderate or severe ventricular dysfunction). Follow-up of an earlier group of aortic valve replacement/coronary artery bypass patients[11] (n=294) identified, by univariate and multivariate analysis, that preoperative age greater or equal to 70 years ($p=0.02$) and Class IV symptoms ($p=0.002$) decreased late survival.

More recently, we have expanded our experience using aortic valve repair for patients with aortic insufficiency.[12] Some of these patients require concomitant coronary artery bypass. Recently, we reviewed our experience with 98 patients who underwent aortic valve repair (unpublished data). Of this group, 27 (28 percent) underwent concomitant coronary artery bypass. When reviewing patients who had undergone aortic valve repair, by univariate analysis, the risks for operative mortality included advanced age, NYHA functional class, etiology and leaflet pathology, and need for additional operation (coronary artery bypass, or other valve operation).

In summary, the combination of valve surgery with coronary artery bypass increases the operative risk beyond that associated with either procedure alone. This increase is seen for all combinations of valve and bypass operations, but is most notable for patients with ischemic mitral regurgitation and ischemic cardiomyopathy. For both mitral and aortic valve operations, the long-term patient outcome is primarily determined by the extent of underlying left ventricular dysfunction and patient age. In general, valve repair is preferable because of a lower operative mortality, and improved long-term survival.

REFERENCES

1. Loop FD: Long-term results of mitral valve repair. Semin Thorac Cardiovasc Surg 1989;1:203–10.
2. Frater RW, Salomon NW, Rainer WG, Cosgrove DM, Wickham E: The Carpentier-Edwards pericardial aortic valve: intermediate results. Ann Thorac Surg 1992;53:764–71.
3. Stewart WJ, Salcedo EE: Echocardiography in patients undergoing mitral valve surgery. Semin Thorac Cardiovasc Surg 1989;1:194–202.
4. Loop FD, Lytle BW, Cosgrove DM, et al: Influence of the internal-mammary-artery graft on 10-year survival and other cardiac events. N Engl Med 1986;314:1–6.
5. Cosgrove DM, Lytle BW, Hill AC, et al: Are two internal thoracic arteries better than one? J Thorac Cardiovasc Surg 1994, in press.
6. Navia D, Cosgrove DM, Lytle BW, et al: Is the internal thoracic artery the conduit of choice to replace a stenotic vein graft? Ann Thorac Surg 1994;57:40–4.
7. Lytle BW, McElroy D, McCarthy PM, et al: Influence of arterial coronary bypass grafts on the mortality in coronary reoperations. J Thorac Cardiovasc Surg 1994;107:675–83.
8. Hendren WG, Nemec JJ, Lytle BW, et al: Mitral valve repair for ischemic mitral insufficiency. Ann Thorac Surg 1991;52:1246–52.
9. Lytle BW, Cosgrove DM, Gill CC, et al: Mitral valve replacement combined with myocardial revascularization: early and late results for 300 patients. Circulation 1985;71:1179–90.
10. Lytle BW, Cosgrove DM, Goormastic M, Loop FD: Aortic valve replacement and coronary bypass grafting for patients with aortic stenosis and coronary artery disease: early and late results. Eur Heart J 1988;9:143–7.
11. Lytle BW, Cosgrove DM, Loop FD, et al: Replacement of aortic valve combined with myocardial revascularization: determinants of early and late risk for 500 patients, 1967–1981. Circulation 1983;68:1149–62.
12. Cosgrove DM, Rosengkranz ER, Hendren WG, Barlett JC, Stewart WJ: Valvuloplasty for aortic insufficiency. Ann Thorac Surg 1991;52:1246–52.

FAILED PTCA: MYOCARDIAL PROTECTION AND SURGICAL MANAGEMENT IN THE CATHETERIZATION LABORATORY

Timothy J. Gardner, M.D.

Hospital of the University of Pennsylvania
Philadelphia, Pennsylvania

Percutaneous transluminal coronary angioplasty (PTCA) has become, for many patients with symptomatic coronary artery obstructive disease, the first and only interventional treatment required to successfully manage their symptomatic state and functional limitations. Intra-arterial angioplasty techniques, first developed for the management of peripheral arterial disease, were introduced into general clinical use for coronary artery disease in the early 1980's and, since that time, have surpassed coronary artery bypass grafting in terms of annual numbers of procedures performed.[1] The appropriate role of coronary angioplasty versus surgical bypass grafting for symptomatic patients with multi-vessel coronary artery disease is currently the subject of several randomized multi-institutional trials and initial information from these trials support the continued, if not expanded, application of PTCA for some patients with multi-vessel coronary artery disease. Because of the potential for the iatrogenic induction of cardiac ischemia and hemodynamic instability, so-called *surgical back-up* has been a feature of virtually all PTCA programs since the initiation of this therapy.[2] At least 5 percent of patients who undergo a PTCA procedure require early surgery, often urgently or emergently undertaken because of the occurrence of myocardial ischemia in the catheterization laboratory.[3] The subject of this review is to present our view on how to best deal with these PTCA failures and whether there is a role for myocardial protective interventions while the patient is in the catheterization laboratory and prior to surgery.

INDICATIONS FOR PTCA

In general, the indications for considering PTCA in any given patient are similar or identical to clinical indications for coronary artery bypass grafting, that is, the presence of myocardial ischemia which is inadequately managed by medical treatment alone. For most patients, this translates to symptomatic coronary artery disease which is unresponsive to or poorly controlled by medical therapy and lifestyle change. For other patients, the presenting evidence of myocardial ischemia may be rest angina or crescendo angina necessitating hospitalization, and for others who are either asymptomatic or only mildly so, ischemia is demonstrable through exercise testing using EKG monitoring or blood flow scanning. The major caveat or determinant for the appropriateness of PTCA, however, will be the suitability of the coronary arterial blockages for percutaneous balloon dilatation or atherectomy.

Common contraindications to PTCA include high risk patterns of coronary artery disease, such as left main coronary artery obstruction or the presence of complex coronary lesions, such as those which span a bifurcation point in a major arterial system, in which case balloon dilation might open the major artery but occlude a secondary branch. Left main coronary artery obstruction, in general, precludes percutaneous dilation or atherectomy because even transient occlusion of this artery is not tolerated. PTCA would be contraindicated also in a situation in which there is a high degree of *myocardial jeopardy* associated with dilation of a particular lesion. A patient with a tight lesion of the very proximal left anterior descending (LAD) coronary artery who has a pre-existing total right coronary artery occlusion and obstructive disease in the circumflex system can be expected to sustain severe myocardial ischemia and hemodynamic instability if the LAD occludes as a result of the PTCA. In situations such as these, angioplasty would be relatively contraindicated. Another contraindication to PTCA is the presence of distal aorto-ileo-femoral occlusive disease, which, if severe, will preclude angioplasty in almost all instances. The brachial artery approach for cannulation of the coronary arteries, although frequently adequate for catheter positioning for coronary angiography, is rarely adequate to allow for insertion and manipulation of an angioplasty catheter.

PTCA COMPLICATIONS

The primary cause of PTCA failure is acute occlusion of the target vessel. Occlusion can be a result of guidewire placement in which the wire dissects into the obstructing plaque, displacing it into the lumen of the artery with abrupt cessation of blood flow and thrombus formation. Guidewire lacerations of the coronary arterial wall, including the left main coronary artery, may also result in a vessel wall dissection with complete or partial occlusion of the artery. Intimal artery wall dissections can also occur from the fracturing action of the dilating balloon catheter with the result that there is a loose intimal disruption which either transiently or recurrently occludes the true lumen of the coronary artery or may actually spiral down to a tight point of blockage.

Other methods of arterial obstruction include rupture of an atheromatous plaque with embolization distally of the plaque content, including lipid globules and calcium. Another form of injury is a mural hematoma at the site of intimal rupture from dilatation. Other technical complications of the PTCA which do not result in acute worsening of the patient's status but nonetheless represent a failure of the therapeutic goal of the angioplasty include inability to cross the lesion with the guidewire, eliminating the possibility of positioning a dilating balloon catheter. Likewise, some lesions will not dilate under even high dilatation pressures. This appears to be the case occasionally in patients with heavily calcified, circumferential coronary arterial blockages.

Finally, one of the major problems associated with PTCA is the likelihood of restenosis of the dilated coronary artery with recurrence of cardiac symptoms. Whether the restenosis is the result of vessel wall recoil or represents a pathological response to localized arterial wall trauma remains to be clarified. It is likely that both factors play a role in restenosis which occurs in as many as 30 percent of patients within one year after PTCA.[4]

PTCA TECHNIQUES

The usual method of percutaneous angioplasty involves dilatation of the arterial obstruction with a pressurized balloon catheter. As noted above, after delineating the coronary artery anatomy and identifying target lesions for dilatation, a fine guidewire is placed across the obstruction and a balloon dilatation catheter is threaded into place over the guidewire. The balloon is then inflated under substantial pressure with dilatation force exceeding several atmospheres. The duration of balloon inflation is, in part, determined by the development of signs of ischemia such as chest pain, EKG changes or bradycardia. The effectiveness of the balloon dilation may be related to the length of time that the vessel wall is compressed with the balloon inflated. On the other hand, it may be possible to achieve satisfactory dilatation by repeated short-duration inflations. Also, it is possible to establish perfusion through the central lumen of the angioplasty catheter into the distal arterial bed with blood or an oxygenated perfluorocarbon solution during protracted inflations to enhance the patient's tolerance to the induced ischemia.

Other techniques for angioplasty under evaluation include the use of so-called *atherectomy techniques* in which a rotating cutting core is used to shave off atherosclerotic material in the obstruction. There are a variety of catheters which have been developed for this purpose, almost all of which share the common risk of arterial wall perforation due to malpositioning of the catheter. There is also the likelihood of some distal arterial embolization of the obstructing plaque material. A variety of new laser catheters are in development which can coagulate the intraluminal obstructions and may be applicable for some patients.

RESULTS OF PTCA

The acute failures of PTCA which require immediate surgery because of impending or evolving myocardial infarction occur somewhere between 2 and 3 percent of cases, based on much of the published material available. A significantly higher proportion of the population undergoing angioplasty, up to 10 percent, will be referred for coronary artery bypass grafting on the same admission because of failure to adequately dilate the obstruction. Acute myocardial infarction occurs in 2 or 3 percent of patients having PTCA and procedure-related deaths occur in slightly more than 1 percent of patients in large PTCA series[3].

On the other hand, the incidence of incomplete revascularization and recurrent angina is quite high. Approximately 30 percent of patients will develop artery restenosis within the first year and many of these patients will be referred for coronary bypass grafting because of progressive or worsening chest pain. Altogether, about one third of patients will require repeat PTCA within three years.

SURGICAL SUPPORT FOR PTCA

Although cardiac catheterizations can be performed in hospitals without on-site cardiac surgical capabilities, this is not the case for interventional catheterization laboratory procedures such as PTCA. Even though the risk of cardiovascular collapse as a result of a PTCA-induced coronary artery obstruction is low, an immediate response to such an event necessitates on-site cardiac surgery support. As a general rule, it should be possible to have the patient who experiences an acute angioplasty failure in the operating room and ready to undergo open heart surgery within one hour from the time the decision is made for surgery. In many large medical centers with large surgical suites, operating room availability may be such that it is not necessary to hold open an operating room to provide availability in the case of an angioplasty failure. In other settings, however, surgical and OR stand-by necessitates a dedicated operating room team with a vacant room to provide for an appropriate response.

An important and useful measure to insure a proper level of readiness on the part of the surgical team is to have the angioplasty operator review multi-vessel or high risk angioplasty patients with the consultant surgeon who can then provide for a heightened level of preparedness under these circumstances.

Specific measures which should be employed in the angioplasty suite to insure effective surgical back-up and intervention when required include the on-site availability of an intra-aortic balloon pump. An additional support technique which should be considered for deployment is the use of so-called *peripheral cardiopulmonary bypass*. This involves the institution of full cardiopulmonary bypass via peripheral arterial and venous cannulation, generally through the femoral artery and vein with connection to a portable bypass apparatus. The availability of hemodynamically efficient cannulae suitable for femoral artery and vein insertion and capable of allowing pump flows in excess of four liters per minute coupled with an efficient membrane oxygenator allows for effective temporary support of a patient who sustains a cardiac arrest or has acute left heart failure. Although there is a significant risk of left ventricular distention should the heart fibrillate or the LV fail to contract in the face of aortic valve incompetence, maintenance of normothermia by a circuit heat exchanger and rapid defibrillation will usually avoid this troublesome complication of peripheral bypass. The other feature of catheterization laboratory readiness which must be insured in order to adequately use either the intra-aortic balloon pump and especially the peripheral bypass system is the availability of a trained perfusionist who can assist the catheterization laboratory team and the surgical consultants in initiating peripheral bypass promptly.

An additional aspect of catheterization laboratory preparedness for such an abrupt hemodynamic collapse is to insure bilateral femoral artery and vein access in order that intra-aortic balloon pump support or even peripheral bypass can be undertaken through one femoral area while the aortic catheter and temporary right heart pacing wire, if indicated, can be maintained and manipulated through the contralateral femoral artery and vein. In high risk patients, it may be advisable to place femoral artery and vein guidewires prior to initiating the PTCA maneuver via the contralateral femoral artery.

TECHNIQUES TO PROTECT THE HEART AFTER FAILED PTCA

In addition to providing for the appropriate organization of the standby team and facilities, and despite having provided for hemodynamic and even circulatory support of the patient who sustains a failed angioplasty and must be taken to surgery immediately, the other crucial ingredient in successful salvage of such a patient involves protecting the heart from irreversible ischemic damage associated with the PTCA induced coronary artery occlusion. Almost all acute angioplasty failures which result in hemodynamic instability are the result of an abrupt complete occlusion of a coronary artery. This clinical circumstance is identical to that associated with an acute occlusion of a coronary artery from a thrombus or embolus. If the artery is not reopened and myocardial blood flow restored very quickly, myocardial infarction and cellular necrosis inevitably occur. The time course of myocardial infarction, as has been established experimentally and clinically, is very rapid with an immediate loss of contractile function in the ischemic region progressing rapidly to extensive myocardial cell necrosis in the region-at-risk. Experimental studies, in animals with few preformed coronary collateral channels, have demonstrated completion of the infarction within 90 to 120 minutes and with as much as 80 percent of the myocardial region-at-risk becoming necrotic.[5] Although this time course may be slower and the extent of infarction less in humans with chronic coronary atherosclerosis, the infarction process will begin very quickly after an interruption of myocardial blood flow and will evolve rapidly.

Techniques available to the angioplasty operator to restore myocardial blood flow after the occurrence of an acute occlusion vary significantly. If the occlusion is the result of a spiraling intimal dissection, it is sometimes possible to compress the false channel by repeat dilatation sufficiently effectively to avoid recurrent obstruction. The availability of detachable stents which hold the coronary artery open after dilatation may also be helpful in *tacking up* the dissected artery wall. If the occlusion is more localized and is the result of plaque dislodgement, direct arterial wall injury or arterial wall hematoma, it may not be possible to keep the artery from re-occluding even after multiple repeat dilatations. In this instance, placement of a catheter with a central lumen which allows for blood flow from above to the area distal to the obstruction, a so-called *bail out* catheter, may be highly effective in maintaining some blood flow past the point of obstruction.[6,7] A general requirement for placing the bail out catheter is the ability to recross the area of obstruction with a guidewire which may not be possible if the angioplasty catheter has been removed prior to occurrence of the complete occlusion. In this latter instance the only option available for establishing blood flow into the myocardium subserved by the obstructed artery is through coronary sinus cannulation.

Despite the fact that coronary sinus perfusion or counter pulsation techniques have been shown to be highly effective in attenuating ischemia in the face of acute coronary occlusions experimentally, these techniques have not been widely adopted clinically, at least in part, because of the logistical challenges of cannulating the coronary sinus in the face of patient instability after an acute coronary occlusion.

Other measures to reduce myocardial oxygen demand and reduce the extent of myocardial ischemic injury in this setting, as the patient is being prepared for emergent transfer to the operating room, is placement of an intra-aortic balloon pump catheter. The diastolic counter pulsation afforded by this technique not only unloads the left ventricle and reduces ventricular work demands but may enhance collateral coronary blood flow by increasing diastolic pressure in the aortic root. In addition, institution of peripheral bypass with volume unloading of the left ventricle as well will further reduce myocardial oxygen demands. The institution of peripheral bypass, however, has the same logistical disadvantages as coronary sinus cannulation techniques, namely a need to devote several additional minutes to instrumenting the patient and initiating the system, an expenditure of time which can be avoided if the patient is taken directly to the operating room. On a strictly operational level, it is frequently at this point in a case of PTCA failure that the direct involvement of the cardiac surgeon is most critical in dealing promptly and expeditiously with the emergency created by the acute coronary artery occlusion. The surgeon should come to the catheterization laboratory and personally assess the situation and the immediacy of the need for transport to the operating room, the level of instability of the patient's condition, and the need for peripheral bypass support. A common error made at this junction in a PTCA complication is for the angioplasty team to persist in trying to reopen an occluded artery beyond a prudent length of time. If the surgical team is not on hand nor readily available, the tendency is to persist longer in what is often a futile effort to reopen an occluded artery. If, however, the surgeon is available in the catheterization laboratory and quickly assumes responsibility for management of the patient, as is appropriate in this situation, the timely decision to take the patient to the operating room and perform surgical revascularization will be enhanced.

OR MANAGEMENT OF THE FAILED PTCA PATIENT

After transporting the patient to the operating room expeditiously, with or without circulatory support, the patient with an acute coronary occlusion and persistent ischemia should be rapidly anesthetized and prepared for placement on central cardiopulmonary bypass. The actual induction of anesthesia is a risky period in which it is possible to induce ischemia-related ventricular arrhythmias. There must be expeditious and skilled management at this time, emphasizing the importance of having the anesthesia team available as well during angioplasty. An anesthesia group which is not experienced in dealing with cardiac surgical patients, especially patients ongoing acute ischemia, will not do as well in this situation as will experienced cardiac anesthesiologists.

The primary goal at this time should be to get the patient on bypass through central cannulation and to initiate the appropriate operative myocardial protective techniques. One useful approach is to commence bypass and to induce systemic hypothermia, to clamp the distal ascending aorta and to arrest the heart, with additional myocardial protection during the ischemic interval achieved by direct topical cardiac cooling. If the patient is relatively young and if the left anterior descending coronary artery requires grafting, it may be reasonable to harvest the left internal mammary artery as a pedicle graft with the patient on bypass, with the aorta cross-clamped and the heart arrested. The safety of this maneuver is based on the demonstrated effectiveness of the myocardial protective strategies used during induced global myocardial ischemia.

If a bail-out catheter was placed through the area of coronary artery obstruction while the patient was in the catheterization laboratory, this catheter must be removed at the time the aorta is cross-clamped. Access to the groin cannulation site should be secured when preparing the patient for surgery. Likewise, if the patient arrives in the operating room on peripheral bypass with cannulation through the groin, once the sternum is divided and the pericardium opened, central cannulae should be placed and the peripheral cannulae removed.

EXPECTED OUTCOME FOLLOWING FAILED PTCA

Virtually all procedure-related mortalities from PTCA occur in patients who have iatrogenic coronary artery occlusions during attempted angioplasty. Despite all of the support and cardiac protective strategies described above, the degree of myocardial injury resulting from the acute coronary occlusion may be so severe that even effective surgical revascularization will not restore cardiac function. On the other hand, since the failed PTCA patient will have suffered a procedure-induced myocardial infarction and since cardiogenic shock which develops early after infarction may resolve, it may be appropriate to continue external ventricular assistance for several days after the surgical procedure with the hope that the degree of cardiac failure will reverse as myocardial stunning abates. The expectation for recovery is especially reasonable if prompt and effective revascularization was achieved by timely coronary artery bypass grafting.

Nonetheless, the mortality for patients who require emergency operation after a failed PTCA exceeds 5 percent. In addition, as many as a third of these patients will have evidence, by electrocardiogram, of having sustained a significant myocardial infarction in association with the angioplasty failure and coronary bypass grafting procedure.[8,9]

REFERENCES

1. Gruentzig AR, Senning A, Siegenthaler WE: Nonoperative dilatation of coronary artery stenosis: percutaneous transluminal coronary angioplasty. N Engl J Med 1979;301:62.
2. Cameron DE, Stinson DC, Greene PS, Gardner TJ: Surgical standby for percutaneous transluminal coronary angioplasty: a survey of patterns of practice. Ann Thorac Surg 1990;50:35–39.
3. Kent KM, Bentivoglio LG, Block PC, et al: PTCA: Report from the Registry of the National Heart, Lung and Blood Institute. Am J Cardiol 1982;49:2011.
4. Jutzy KR, Berte LE, Alderman EL, et al: Coronary restenosis rates in consecutive patient series one year post successful angioplasty. Circulation 1982;66(Suppl II):II-331.
5. Homeffer PJ, Healy B, Gott VL, Gardner TJ: The rapid evolution of a myocardial infarction in an end-artery coronary preparation. Circulation 1987;76(Suppl V):V-39.
6. Turi ZG, Campbell CA, Gottimukkala MV, Kloner RA: Preservation of distal coronary perfusion with an autoperfusion angioplasty catheter. Circulation 1987;75:1273–1280.
7. Angelini P, Leachman R, Heibig J: Distal coronary hemoperfusion during balloon angioplasty. Cardiology 1988;5:13–34.
8. Parsonet V, Fisch D, Gielchinsky I, et al: Emergency operation after failed angioplasty. J Thorac Cardiovasc Surg 1988;96:198–203.
9. Golding LAR, Loop FD, Hollman JL, et al: Early results of emergency surgery after coronary angioplasty. Circulation 1986;74(Suppl 3):26–29.

TREATMENT OF ACUTE THORACIC AORTIC DISSECTIONS

Jan D. Galla, M.D. and Randall B. Griepp, M.D.

Mount Sinai Medical Center
New York, New York 10029

INTRODUCTION

Despite the ever-increasing awareness of disorders of the thoracic aorta, these diseases remain among the most frightening conditions for those physicians who do not routinely deal with them. Included within this broad category are aneurysms, thromboses, and the various inflammatory states, but perhaps none of these generate the anxiety evoked by the diagnosis of aortic dissection. Although recent advances in the preoperative recognition and management, intraoperative techniques, and long term follow up and control have greatly increased the survival of these patients, for the majority of physicians this group of diagnoses remains a mysterious and confounding entity. This discussion will attempt to briefly describe these conditions in their acute phase, along with the different approaches, both medically and operatively that have been adopted in our institution. Our experience over the period 1985–1992 will be presented.

BACKGROUND

The thoracic aorta is a question mark shaped structure arising from the aortic valve annulus, extending cephalad into the superior mediastinum before arcing laterally and posterior. It then continues caudad along the thoracic spine and esophagus to the diaphragmatic hiatus, where it enters the abdomen and continues in the retroperitoneum until it bifurcates into the two iliac arteries in the pelvis.

Within the thorax, the aorta is divided into three segments, the ascending, the transverse, and the descending aortas. Several classifications of aortic dissections have been devised, among the earliest of which is the DeBakey system that describes 3 different forms.[1] More recently, in an effort to correlate anatomy with outcome, the Stanford classification has been proposed and has found great acceptance in the literature.[2] In this latter scheme, all thoracic dissections are grouped into two categories, type A or type B, depending only on whether the ascending aorta is involved. The intimal tear may therefore be in the ascending aorta, or either the aortic arch or descending aorta with retrograde extension into the ascending segment for the dissection to be categorized as a type A. Type B dissections, on the other hand, are limited to the aorta distad to the left subclavian artery, but may extend into the abdominal aorta and further. Additionally, the initial intimal tear may arise in the lower thorax or abdomen and propagate in a retrograde direction to the subclavian artery and still be classed as a type B dissection.

The results of management of thoracic dissections have been found to closely parallel their classification based on the Stanford scheme. Type A dissections are virtually 100 percent lethal, with the majority of deaths occurring within the first two weeks, while type B dissections often develop into a chronic form that may last for several years before rupture. Table 1 demonstrates the relative frequencies of these two types of dissections as well as the causes of death for each, if treated solely by medical means. It can be readily seen that not only do type A dissections occur more frequently than those limited to the descending aorta, but cause of death is more sudden and usually related to intrapericardial rupture. Type B dissections usually affect other organ systems by involvement of their arterial supplies, with rupture occurring less frequently. Thus, it may be seen that the type A dissections constitute a more emergent category of disease, requiring rapid diagnosis and initiation of surgical therapy.

Diagnosis of aortic dissection demands a high index of suspicion in patients complaining of acute onset of thoracic pain, especially if accompanied by a history of hypertension. Associated clinical findings are varied and may include syncope, asymmetric or absent pulses, new murmurs, neurological disturbances, renal or intestinal infarction, or myocardial infarction. Definitive diagnosis is made by any of a variety of radiological techniques, including computed tomography (CT), magnetic resonance imaging (MRI), aortography, or transesophageal echocardiography (TEE). Each of these modalities has its advantages and proponents. In our patients, the diagnosis is usually initially made by CT scan, either at our institution or having been sent with the patient from the referring hospital. Our preference is to ascertain the presence of ascending aortic involvement by TEE, reserving

Table 1. Causes of Death in Medically Treated Acute Dissection

Type A		75%
	Rupture	80%
	Heart failure secondary to aortic insufficiency	10%
	Branch obstruction	10%
Type B		15%
	Rupture	30%
	Branch obstruction	70%

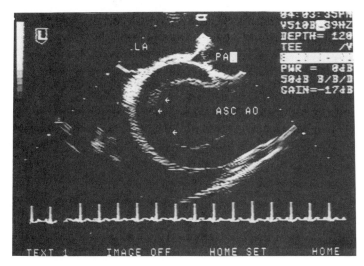

Figure 1. Echocardiographic appearance of an ascending aortic dissection. LA = left atrium; PA = pulmonary artery; ASC AO = ascending aorta. Intimal flap with tears is indicated by white arrow.

aortography for those patients in whom TEE is contraindicated or in whom the diagnosis remains unclear after TEE. The typical TEE appearance of an ascending aortic dissection is seen in Figure 1. If an ascending dissection is seen by TEE, diagnosis of type A dissection is confirmed and the patient is prepared for urgent surgery. Those patients in whom an ascending dissection is not seen are treated with an aggressive medical approach based upon heart rate and blood pressure control unless operative criteria are met. These criteria include failure of medical therapy (as evidenced by persistent pain or intractable hypertension), left hemothorax, or lower limb ischemia.

The following data are derived from those patients with acute thoracic aortic dissections requiring surgery during the period 1985–1992.

MATERIALS AND METHODS

Patients

Sixty four patients with acute aortic dissection during the period 1985–1992 required surgery. Of these, 52 were type A dissections and the remainder (12) were type B. Patient characteristics are listed in Table 2. Males predominated in the type A group but near equality of sexes was seen in the type B patients. The type A patients tended to be somewhat younger although the age range was similar in the two groups. None of the type B patients demonstrated either neurologic or hemodynamic compromise prior to surgery, conditions that were seen in approximately 20 percent of the type A patients. Also included within the type A group were three (3) Marfan's disease patients.

Table 2. Acute Dissection Patient Population

	Type A (n=52)	Type B (n=12)
Male/female	40/12	7/5
Age (range)	55(27–79)	64(54–73)
Marfan syndrome	3	0
Hemodynamic compromise	10	0
New neurological event	11	0

Procedures

All patients underwent replacement of the diseased aortic segments. None of the patients in either type A or type B groups were repaired with the use of gelatinresorcinol glue or other binders.

Of the 52 patients in the type A group, the proximal anastomosis of the ascending aorta was hand sewn in 33 (63%) of the patients. Thirteen (25%) of the patients were repaired with the Bentall procedure. Eleven of these were conducted after the method of Kouchoukos et al.,[3] using coronary artery buttons for reimplantation, while the other 2 patients had involvement of their coronary ostia necessitating the Cabrol modification for reconstruction.[4] The remaining 6 patients were repaired with a proximal intraluminal graft.

In 50 percent of our patients, only the ascending aorta required replacement. In 6 of these patients, the distal anastomosis was performed in a hand-sewn fashion, employing a brief period of circulatory arrest to excise the site of the aortic cross clamp, reconstruct the aorta and perform the anastomosis. Nineteen patients were repaired with an intraluminal graft tied into position just proximal to the origin of the innominate artery.

In the remaining group of type A dissections, reconstruction of the aortic arch was required. A partial *hemi-arch* replacement was required in 13 patients and a complete arch replacement was needed in the rest. Both of these arch procedures were conducted with deep hypothermia and circulatory arrest. The arrest interval varied with the extent of the repair, usually being limited to approximately 15 to 20 minutes for a partial arch and 30 to 45 minutes for a complete arch repair. During these arrest intervals, esophageal temperatures were routinely lowered to 13 to 16°C and the head packed in ice. If prolongation (greater than 30 minutes) of circulatory arrest were anticipated, steroids and barbiturates were administered prior to the period of arrest.

Twelve patients underwent repair of an acute type B dissection. One patient was repaired by simple cross clamping of the aorta, without distal perfusion. Of the remaining 11 patients, 8 were perfused retrograde using the Biomedicus® pump, 2 were repaired under hypothermic circulatory arrest (HCA), and 1 was repaired under partial cardiopulmonary bypass. In all instances, the diseased segment of the aorta was excised entirely and lumbar bleeders were controlled with hemaclips. The 2 patients repaired under HCA were done in that fashion to obtain better proximal tissue to use for the anastomosis. Cerebral perfusion was reinitiated after completion of the proximal anastomosis by clamping the distal end of the graft and inserting the arterial perfusion cannula into a hole made in the graft material. The circulatory arrest interval was usually 15 to 18 minutes, and pre-arrest steroids and/or barbiturates were not given.

For both type A and B dissection repairs, the graft material was double woven velour, either coated with albumin and baked in the autoclave, or factory prepared collagen impregnated Hemashield grafts. The distal segments of the aorta were visually inspected prior to completion of the anastomoses to insure the intimal tear was resected with the specimen and no secondary tears were evident. Aortic wall integrity was reconstituted by sandwiching the two dissected layers between Teflon felt and either felt or pericardium on the inside of the aorta, using a simple running 3-0 or 4-0 polypropylene suture. We firmly believe that this sandwiching technique prior to the graft to aorta anastomosis helps to reduce needle hole leaks, either externally or, more importantly, into the false lumen. Anastomoses were created with a second running suture of 3-0 or 4-0 running polypropylene between the graft and the reconstructed aortic wall.

Aortic root reconstructions in the Bentall repairs were performed with interrupted, pledgetted 2-0 Ethibond® sutures (Ethicon Inc., Somerville, NJ), oriented with the pledgets on the aortic side of the annulus. Native aorta was excised from the ascending segment to facilitate exposure and to help in determination of bleeding sites post-repair. Coronary button anastomoses were performed with continuously running 4-0 or 5-0 polypropylene, as were coronary to graft anastomoses in the Cabrol modification. Ten mm graft (either Gortex® or woven velour) was routinely used for this procedure.

Intraluminal grafts were employed for their completeness in obliterating the false lumen more frequently than their ease and rapidity of insertion. These grafts were not only secured at their bases with the double ligatures provided but also wrapped externally about the ligature site with a wide band of Teflon felt.[5]

The routine use of intraoperative TEE allows monitoring of intra-aortic flows in the true and false lumens both at the onset of bypass and at the resumption of reperfusion following intervals of circulatory arrest. This prevents inadvertent perfusion of the false lumen either initially or at a later stage of the procedure.

Postoperative Management

Patients were managed in a routine fashion as postoperative open heart patients in the cardiac surgical intensive unit. Blood pressure and heart rates were controlled with intravenous agents, including β-blocking agents, as necessary. Extubation, chest tube removal and cessation of intravascular monitoring lines were performed as per ICU protocols. Initiation of oral antihypertensive and β-blocking agents was performed as rapidly as possible, as was mobilization of the patient. All patients, prior to their discharge, were urged to undergo repeat aortography and CT scanning. Postoperative echocardiography was limited to those patients that underwent resuspension of their aortic valves to assess residual aortic insufficiency.

Follow-up

All patients were followed through their hospital course for instances of reoperation or death. Mortality was scored as hospital death if death occurred prior to discharge, irrespective of duration of stay. Late deaths were those patients that died subsequent to discharge. Every effort was made to determine cause of death, including autopsy, whenever possible. After discharge, patients were followed by serial CT scans at yearly intervals and by telephone interviews with both patients and their physicians.

RESULTS

Type A Dissections

All type A dissections underwent operative repair. Whenever possible, the native aortic valve was spared by repair or resuspension. Exception to this rule was made for those patients exhibiting annulo-aortic ectasia associated with their dissections (Marfan syndrome). In this group of patients, composite graft repair of the aortic valve and ascending aorta was routinely performed.

The diseased segment of aorta was closely inspected and whenever possible the intimal tear was resected with the specimen. The segment of aorta adjacent to that resected was also carefully inspected whenever possible, especially when circulatory support was interrupted. If additional tears were visualized, attempts were made to include those areas in the resection as well.

Unless a substantial piece of healthy aorta was available proximal to the cross clamp, the distal anastomosis was performed with a brief period of HCA. Despite the need for deep hypothermic conditions and its associated complications, the enhanced visibility of the distal aortic stump allowed exact placement of the distal suture line and therefore a very secure anastomosis.

The operative pathology was noted in all cases (Table 3). The ascending aorta contained the initial tear in 31 cases while in 15 patients the tear was in the arch. An intimal tear was found in both of these segments in 1 patient and a retrograde extension of a type B dissection was found in 5 patients. Although, as indicated above, the aortic valve was spared whenever possible, replacement was required in 25 percent of all type A dissections.

Perfusion data were available for 50 of the type A dissection patients (Table 4). Perfusion characteristics were similar for all of the patients except for that interval of HCA and the esophageal temperature was longer and lower, respectively, for the complete arch repairs. The temperatures were deliberately lowered initially to maximize the protective effect on the brain. The longer arrest interval was required to repair the diseased aorta associated with the great vessels and the subsequent anastomosis of the longer suture line around those vessels. The shortest interval of HCA, as might be expected, was seen in a simple anastomosis of the distal aortic graft. Despite the apparent differences in length of HCA in these three groups, considerable variation in duration of arrest existed within each group. There was no

Table 3. Operative Pathology in Acute Type A Dissections

Site of tear	
Ascending aorta	60%
Aortic arch	29%
Both	2%
Descending aorta	10%
Aortic valve replacement required	25%

Table 4. Perfusion and Hypothermic Circulatory Arrest Parameters for Acute A Dissection Repairs

	CPB (min)	AXC (min)	HCA Duration (min)	Temperature (°C)
Ascending (n=25)	187	102	28(12–66)	16
Partial arch (n=13)	220	114	38(20–54)	14
Complete arch (n=12)	204	88	54(19–80)	11

CPB = cardiopulmonary bypass; AXC = aortic cross-clamp; HCA = hypothermic circulatory arrest

significant difference in either the cross clamp or cardiopulmonary bypass time among the three groups of patients.

There were 10 (19%) hospital deaths, occurring between 0 and 31 days of surgery (Table 5). Multiple organ systems failure occurred in three patients, usually in the early postoperative period. Continued extension of the dissection process within the residual aortic wall causes myocardial infarction in three patients, also early in the postoperative period. One later death from this cause occurred on postoperative day 31. This represented the latest of all in hospital deaths. Other causes of in hospital deaths included a rupture of the descending aorta in one patient, the thrombosis of a Cabrol graft in one patient, and sudden unexplained death in 2 patients. All of these other causes of death occurred at 10 postoperative days.

There were 2 late deaths (Table 6), one resulting from complications of anticoagulation at 1 year after surgery and the other of sudden, unexplained causes at 3 years after surgery. These 2 deaths in the patients

Table 5. Hospital Mortality in Acute Type A Dissection Patients

Cause of death	No. of Patients	Time of Death (days)
Multiple organ failure	3	2, 6, 10
Myocardial infarct due to coronary dissection	3	0, 1, 31
Sudden unexplained	2	10
Ruptured descending aorta	1	10
Thrombosis of Cabrol graf	1	10

Table 6. Late Deaths in Acute Type A Dissection Patients

Cause of death	No. of patients
Anticoagulation complication (1 year)	1
Sudden (3 years)	1

Table 7. Preoperative Factors Which Increase Operative Risk in Patients With Acute Type A Dissections

Risk factors	Discharged patients	Hospital deaths
Coronary dissection	17%	40%
New neurological event	12%	60%
Shock	12%	50%

surviving discharge give an overall late survival of greater than 95 percent (2/42 patients).

An analysis of preoperative factors thought to put the patients at increased risk for surgery found that three events routinely increased mortality for repair of type A dissections. These include involvement of the coronary arteries, preoperative shock or hemodynamic instability, and the presence of a new neurological event. In some patients, more than one of the factors may exist at presentation, with resultant increase in risk. The percentages of these risk factors in both the surviving patients and those dying in the hospital are presented in Table 7.

Three patients required reoperation after their initial procedures (Table 8). One patient, in whom peri-operative hemorrhage was controlled with an aortic wrap and shunt into the right atrium, had a persistent fistula three months postoperatively and began to exhibit signs of right heart overload. He returned and underwent reexploration to suture ligate a bleeding point on the anastomosis. Another patient in whom a valve suspension had been initially performed, developed progressive aortic insufficiency and required valve replacement. The third patient extended his dissection into the abdominal aorta and required fenestration of the aorta for mesenteric and renal artery compromise. The overall incidence of reoperation after type A repair was 2.6 percent/patient year.

Table 8. Reasons for Reoperation Following Acute Type A Dissection Repair*

Procedure at reoperation	No. of patients
Closure of Ao-RA fistula (3 months)	1
Aortic valve replacement (5 months)	1
Fenestration procedure, abdominal aorta (6 months)	1

Ao = aorta; RA = right atrium; *overall incidence 2.6%/patient year.

Type B Dissection

There were no hospital or late deaths in the type B dissection group of patients. There were also no patients with any neurologic sequelae following the repair of their acute dissection. Follow up for periods to 5 years showed no patients returning for reoperation after repair of their dissection. Actuarial survival and freedom from reoperation are therefore 100 percent in this series.

COMMENT

Acute dissection of the thoracic aorta is a disease being discovered with greater frequency as primary care physicians become more cognizant of its presenting symptoms. The rapidity with which the diagnosis may be made has increased tremendously with the advent of relatively noninvasive techniques such as CT scanning, MRI, and echocardiography. The recent application of TEE to the diagnosis of this entity and its acceptance by both the medical and surgical communities as an accurate method of establishing the diagnosis of dissection as well as localizing the intimal tear often obviates the need to undergo more rigorous and invasive intravascular contrast radiological testing.

As the diagnosis of aortic dissection is made more frequently, it is incumbent upon the medical community to establish the optimal method of managing this group of patients. Type A dissections are catastrophic events that may involve the entire length of the aorta to its bifurcation and beyond. The development of appropriate surgical techniques to deal with this condition and its various complications have helped reduce the very high incidence of death.[6] While the degree of lethality is much lower with medical management of type B dissections, authorities are not in agreement that nonoperative management should be the preferred therapy. Convincing arguments exist for early intervention in all dissections, including the initial presentation of type B patients.[7,8] The results presented in this paper would certainly argue that in experienced hands, surgical correction of descending dissections result in minimal morbidity and low mortality, with long lasting, event free results. While those dissections involving the ascending aorta have a much higher operative mortality, the data show that a substantial percentage of this mortality arises from pre-existing factors.

While similar results were obtained in the one instance of simple cross clamping of the aorta and subsequent repair without the use of perfusion or hypothermic circulatory arrest, it is our routine to employ some method of protection of the spinal cord during repair of descending aortic dissections. Other investigators have demonstrated similar event-free results from using the *clamp and cut* method of repair,[9] however, we believe that the uncertainties associated with dissection repairs warrant the effort to provide some form of spinal protection. Among these uncertainties are the extent of the dissection and of the repair, involvement of visceral or spinal arteries, or complications encountered during anatomic dissection (e.g., previous surgery or infection resulting in extensive adhesions or calcifications). We have found the use of retrograde perfusion via the femoral artery to be useful in most of the descending aortic dissections, reserving more complex forms of bypass for those dissections expected to be unusually difficult or extensive. The most frequently used perfusion system is a centrifugal pump (e.g., Biomedicus®, Medtronic Inc., Minneapolis, MN) inserted between the left atrium and the femoral artery. More extensive bypass systems may be initiated via the femoral artery and vein, with supplemental accesses added during the repair. In all repairs utilizing retrograde perfusion, however, it is necessary to insure that flow is not entering a blind channel that could potentially rupture and result in the death of the patient.

The more acute and serious nature of the type A dissection is illustrated by its increased mortality. Despite early, aggressive surgical intervention, almost 20 percent of our patients died of this disease. These deaths most commonly occurred as a result of multiple organ system failure or coronary artery involvement, two well known complications of type A dissections. There were no deaths that could be directly attributed to neurological causes, although 2 patients died of sudden unexplainable causes that may have resulted from extension of the dissection into the cerebral vessels. Additionally, one patient died as a result of continued dissection and subsequent rupture of the descending thoracic aorta, despite what was thought to be an adequate repair at the time of surgery. The only other death resulted from a thrombosed coronary graft.

The problem of persistent patent false lumens after repair has recently been addressed by Ergin et al.[10] In their review of 58 patients undergoing repair of type A dissections, 47 percent of patients that underwent postoperative radiological evaluation were found to have persistent patent false lumens, despite careful attempts to eliminate any observable intimal tears at the time of repair. There was no statistical difference in the number of patients with patent false lumens when those having hand sewn distal anastomoses were compared to those repaired with intraluminal grafts, but antegrade distal lumen flow was not seen in any of the intraluminal graft repaired aortas. Two of the 3 late postoperative deaths occurred in patients with persistent patent distal false lumens and the incidence of complications and reoperations was higher in this group as well. These authors emphasized the need for continued lifelong medical surveillance in patients who have had type A dissections repaired, as well as the need for a sound initial operation to improve their long term prognoses.

We have shown that the use of aggressive preoperative medical management coupled with appropriately timed surgical intervention using sound surgical techniques can lead to long term, event free survival in patients with type B dissections. Despite the increased mortality and complications associated with type A dissections, by using similar principles in the treatment of these patients, we have achieved an acceptable survival and postoperative complication rate for this highly lethal condition. When coupled with our program of long term follow up and life long surveillance, we can offer these patients a reasonable expectation of a continued meaningful life.

REFERENCES

1. DeBakey, ME, Henly, WS, Cooley, DA, et al: Surgical management of dissecting aneurysms of the aorta. J Thorac Cardiovasc Surg 1965;49: 130–149.

2. Daily, PO, Trueblood, HW, Stinson, EB, et al: Management of acute aortic dissections. Ann Thorac Surg 1970;10:237–247.
3. Kouchoukos, NT, Marshall, WG Jr, Wedige-Stecher TA: Eleven-year experience with composite graft replacement of the ascending aorta and aortic valve. J Thorac Cardiovasc Surg 1986;92:691–705.
4. Cabrol C, Pavie A, Mesnildrey P, et al: Long-term results with total replacement of the ascending aorta and reimplantation of the coronary arteries. J Thorac Cardiovasc Surg 1986;91:17–25.
5. Lansman SL, Ergin MA, Galla JD, et al: Intraluminal graft repair of ascending, arch, descending and thoracoabdominal aortic segments for dissecting and aneurysmal disease: long-term follow-up. Semin Thorac Cardiovasc Surg 1991;3:180–182.
6. Masuda Y, Yamada Z, Morooka N, et al: Prognosis of patients with medically treated aortic dissections. Circulation 1991;84(III):7–13.
7. Ergin MA, Galla JD, Lansman S, et al: Acute dissections of the aorta: current surgical treatment. Surg Clin North Am 1985;65:721–741.
8. Svensson LG, Crawford ES: Aortic dissection and aortic aneurysm surgery: Clinical observations, experimental investigations, and statistical analyses part II. Curr Prob Surg 1992;29:917–1057.
9. Mattox KL, Holtzman M, Pickard LR, et al: A safe technique for treatment of blunt injury to the descending thoracic aorta. Ann Thorac Surg 1985;40:456–463.
10. Ergin MA, Phillips RA, Galla JD, et al: Significance of distal false lumen following type A dissection repair. Ann Thorac Surg 1994;57:820–825.

COARCTATION OF THE AORTA: SURGICAL TECHNIQUE AND CONTROVERSIES

Robert B. Karp, M.D.

The University of Chicago
Pritzker School of Medicine
Chicago, Illinois

In late 1944, Craaford, and in 1945, Gross, reported their first cases of surgical repair of coarctation of the aorta. These early cases were done in children using techniques involving resection of the coarcted area and end-to-end anastomosis of the aorta. In 1962, Schuster and Gross reported on 505 cases done at Boston Children's Hospital,[1] 487 of these patients had some sort of resection and end to end anastomosis; occasionally, using interposition of homograft aortic tissue. The mortality in these cases was 4.1 percent. Eighteen patients had exploration without resection. This paper might be considered a landmark one. However, on re-reading in the light of current knowledge and concerns, the paper lacks numerical accuracy. It does not identify with any precision the median age of patients nor age ranges of patients operated upon. It is lacking somewhat in the description of complications or mode of death, and certainly does not approach the problem of inadequate treatment of coarctation or recurrence of the coarctation or late stenosis at the anastomotic site. Nevertheless, the operative survival is remarkable.

For a long while, the teaching (as expounded by Gross's group) was to postpone operation until the age of between five and ten years, with the aim of having larger structures and easier access. What has become apparent in all aspects of congenital heart surgery is that during the waiting period, whether it be one month for an atrial switch or five years for coarctation repair, there may be a large nonsurgical (medical) mortality. Thus, today we look at survivorship in congenital heart disease as one that includes all patients admitted to the institution, generally reflecting mortality figures from day of birth onward. Thus, it becomes imperative to move operation closer and closer within the neonatal period.

Perhaps the controversies in the treatment of coarctation were crystallized in a paper by Bergdahl et.al.[2] from the University of Alabama. In that study, they compared two techniques of coarctation repair in patients aged less than one year operated on between 1967 and 1981. Waldhausen earlier had described the subclavian flap technique which was a variation of the Blalock-Park technique previously used at John Hopkins.[3] In essence, this patches open the area of the coarctation, and alleviates the need for a tiny anastomosis in a small subject using the end to end technique. In the Bergdahl paper using the end to end technique, 13 of 21 patients died for 62 percent mortality. Using the subclavian flap technique, only 2 of 30 patients died for a 7 percent mortality. The authors suggested that the later technique achieved better results in terms of mortality and long-term lack of recoarctation. This paper stimulated a lively debate, and has resulted in comparisons over the subsequent years between generally three types of coarctation repair in the neonate.

The subclavian flap arterioplasty has been used by us and others for about 15 years. Perhaps it is best applied in those patients less than age one year because it does sacrifice the left subclavian artery, and does result in very minimal, but sometimes noticeable growth changes in the left upper extremity. There have been one or two reported cases of major ischemic changes after sacrifice of the left subclavian artery, either for the subclavian flap arterioplasty or for a classic Blalock-Taussig shunt. It has been our practice to leave intact the vertebral, mammary, and thyrocervical branches of the remaining subclavian artery. In any event, the aorta is exposed, and clamps are placed proximal to the coarctation across the transverse aorta between the left carotid and subclavian artery, and distally well below the coarctation, but at an angle to allow intercostal flow. The PDA is ligated. The subclavian artery is ligated or occluded with a hemaclip just proximal to its trifurcation, and incised such as to bring the incision anterolaterally across the isthmus of the aorta and extending across the coarctation onto the descending aorta some 8–12 mm below the coarcted area. When visible, the coarctation membrane is superficially resected, taking care not to remove a great deal of posterior intima. The resulting flap of subclavian artery is then folded down across this vertical incision, and the resulting two sides of the subclavian flap are sutured to the aorta using fine polyprophylene suture. This procedure is generally quite a straight forward operative technique, but is not useful in some of the situations where there is major isthmic hypoplasia. In that case, a variation of the classic end to end anastomosis is performed, generally referred to as an extended or radical end to end anastomosis. The aorta is isolated as usual, carrying the dissection proximally to the innominate artery, well mobilizing the descending aorta, and ligating the ductus arteriosus. A spoon shape or Dera clamp is used to occlude the proximal aorta, the proximal extent of the occlusion being just distal to the takeoff of the innominate artery. The descending aorta is also occluded and the area of coarctation resected in such a way as to have the proximal resection reach well under the origin of the left carotid artery. Often, the distal end of the aorta is spatulated laterally, and the aorta is moved up to approximate the rather long incision in the transverse and isthmic aorta where an end to end anastomosis is made, generally using fine continuous suture.

A third approach to repair of coarctation of the aorta in both neonates and older patients is the use of a simple patch graft. This is particularly appropriate for reoperations on the aorta, and in patients who are older having accompanying degenerative changes of the aortic tissue. In this procedure, the aorta is again exposed, but not fully mobilized posteriorly. Clamps are placed across the isthmus between the left carotid and left subclavian, and well below the area of coarctation. The key to this operation is the use of a rather wide, almost diamond shaped patch to close this defect. The widest part of the patch, of course, bridges the area of coarctation, and the Dacron or Goretex patch should bulge at the conclusion of the procedure. The patch is inserted with polyethylene suture as in the previous techniques. Associated with this procedure has been an incidence of aneurysmal dilatation of the native aortic tissue posteriorly. This probably is attributable to two factors. One is excessive resection of the coarction diaphragm before placement of the patch, and also to the differences in compliance characteristics of the native tissue and the patch material.

In addition to the type of surgical repair, there are several other influences on survivorship after coarctation repair in the young subject. In patients with isolated coarctation and without ventricular septal defect or major associated cardiac defects, the results are best. The addition of a ventricular septal defect to the complex increases mortality. Mortality is highest in those patients with major associated defects other than isolated ventricular septal defect such as Taussig-Bing abnormality, double outlet right ventricle, and so on. It has been noted that the classic description of coarctation of the aorta, that is a membrane juxtaposed to the origin of the ductus arteriosus producing an isolated narrowing, is rare and is a flawed concept. In most cases, there is some associated narrowing of the aorta between the origin of the left subclavian artery and the ligamentum. This area is referred to as the isthmus, and many coarctations have isthmic hypoplasia. In addition, the transverse arch often is somewhat narrowed. Besides the complexity of the total congenital malformation and the anatomy of the area related to the coarctation, the age and weight of the patient have been found to be related to operative risk.

We have recently examined the results of coarctation repair in our pediatric population over the past seven years. Seventy-three patients were operated upon, and six died with a mortality of 8.2 percent (confidence limits 4.9–13.0 percent). Thirty patients less than age one month were operated upon, and there were five deaths for 16.7 percent mortality (confidence limits 9.5–26.7 percent). Thirteen patients one to three months were operated upon with one death and a 7.7 percent mortality (confidence limits 1.0–23.8 percent). Thirty patients older than three months were operated upon with no deaths. In addition to the effect of age on operative mortality, the complexity of the underlying malformation influenced mortality. For example, in those with simple isolated coarctation, there were 38 patients with no deaths. In those with ventricular septal defect, there were 17 patients with ultimately two patients dying and in those with more complex malformations, there were 18 patients with four deaths. The six deaths in this group were generally patients either awaiting a second procedure, or during the second or third operation for a more complex malformation. The technique of operation varied among the group.

Twenty-one patients had subclavian flap angioplasty, 28 patients had end to end or radical end to end anastomosis, and 20 patients had patch angioplasty with four others having a tube graft. The mortality among those groups did not differ.

Recently, there has been great interest in the anatomic malformations associated with coarctation of the aorta. Thus, coarctation as an entity may be seen as a spectrum, varying between an isolated obstruction at the juxtaductal area, to variations of the hypoplastic left heart syndrome. The group at Boston Children's and others have begun to look at coarctation as part of a left heart aorta complex. Kirklin and others as members of a multi-institutional study group associated with the Congenital Heart Surgeons Society have collected information among 25 institutions on the anatomy and results associated with operation for variations of the left heart aorta complex.[4] The left heart aorta complex may be classified into four classes. Class I includes coarctation (or interrupted aortic arch) or any other one obstructive anomaly in one area of the left heart aorta complex including mitral stenosis or its variants, reduced left ventricular size, narrowing of the left ventricular outflow tract, or hypoplasia of the ascending aorta. Thus coarctation is only one of the factors in left heart aorta complex. HLH class II includes coarctation plus mitral valve abnormalities or other hypoplastic ascending aorta complexes. Class III includes abnormalities in three areas, usually including left ventricular hypoplasia, coarctation or isthmic narrowing, and left ventricular outflow tract narrowing. Class IV is the usual hypoplastic left heart syndrome, that is abnormalities in four areas, usually including mitral atresia or narrowing, small left ventricular cavity, left ventricular outflow tract obstruction, and aortic atresia. Of interest class II, III, and IV may each constitute hypoplastic left heart syndrome (not isolated coarctation), but at times may not always require an ultimate single ventricle operation.

When we looked at those 73 infants and retrospectively classified them as to their hypoplastic left heart class, 64 patients were class I, and there were four deaths. Five patients were class II, and there was one death, and four patients were class III and there was one death. Thus, a further obvious but now refined method of classifying incremental risk for coarctation repair lies in the classification of hypoplastic left heart syndrome.

Preliminary results from the above noted Congenital Heart Surgeons Society study of coarctation and related malformations might clarify some of these distinctions. In a two year period, 169 neonates having coarctation without ventricular septal defect underwent some intervention in the 25 hospitals included in this study. One hundred forty-five patients had coarctation only, and there were six total deaths (4 percent, confidence limit 2–7 percent). There were 12 patients having hypoplastic left heart class II. There were six deaths. There were 12 additional patients having two or more additional left heart aorta anomalies (class III) and there were ten deaths in that group. When the group was enlarged by including those both with and without ventricular septal defect, (n=322) specific incremental risk factors for death emerged. Basically, lower age at repair and multiplicity of ventricular septal defects increased the hazard for early death. Additional incremental risk factors were larger size of ventricular septal defect, mitral valve anomaly, subaortic narrowing, aortic valve stenosis, left ventricular hypoplasia, and associated severe non-cardiac anomalies. Among the 169 patients without ventricular septal defects, the type of operation had no clear superiority in terms of survivorship. For instance, 68 patients with end to end anastomosis were included, and there were 9 deaths (13 percent mortality, confidence limits 9–19 percent). These subclavian flap operations were used in 69 patients in whom there were 5 deaths (7 percent mortality, confidence limits 4–12 percent). Patch graft angioplasty was used in 17 patients in whom there were 3 deaths (17 percent mortality, confidence limits 8–32 percent).

What we have learned about coarctation is that operation should be undertaken soon in the neonatal period if the patient is symptomatic. Otherwise, the patient will die without an operation. However, lower age and lower birth weight of the patient affect results. The complexity of the associated congenital malformation certainly affects the results, but the technique of operation seems not to affect survivorship

REFERENCES

1. Schuster SR, Gross RE: Surgery for coarctation of the aorta. A review of 500 cases. J Thorac Cardiovasc Surg 1962;43:54–70.
2. Bergdahl LA, Blackstone EH, Kirklin JW, Pacifico AD, Bargeron LM Jr: Determinants of early success in repair of aortic coarctation in infants. J Thorac Cardiovasc Surg 1982;83(5):736–742.
3. Waldhausen JA, Nahrwald DL: Repair of coarctation of the aorta with a subclavian flap. J Thorac Cardiovasc Surg 1966;51:532–540.
4. Quaegebur J, Jonas R, Weinberg et al: Outcomes in seriously ill neonates with coarctation of the aorta: a multi-institutional study. J Thorac Cardiovasc Surg 1994, to be published.

SELECTION OF CONDUITS FOR PRIMARY AND RE-DO OPERATIONS

John L. Ochsner, M.D.

Ochsner Clinic
New Orleans, LA

Selection of conduits for coronary bypass operation is not any different for a primary than for a re-operation for myocardial revascularization. However, in re-operations, the availability of conduit is likely to be the most important factor in selection since use of multiple grafts in an earlier operation or operations may greatly limit the surgeon's options. Many other factors besides availability of conduit determine the selection of a conduit, including:

1. *Size of myocardial bed.* One should not expect a conduit of small diameter to supply a large mass of myocardium, which normally requires more flow than is possible from the new smaller graft.
2. *Expected longevity of patient.* It is not necessary to utilize a conduit, which has proven long-term patency in a patient whose expected longevity is short.
3. *Coagulation status of patient.* When a patient is transferred to surgery from having undergone treatment with thrombolytic drugs, it is unwise and dangerous to dissect out arteries from which there might be considerable bleeding from the dissected area because of a coagulation defect.
4. *Urgency of revascularization.* Where revascularization is urgent, such as following an acute myocardial infarction, the quickest manner in which one can supply blood to the infarcted area, the less chance for permanent damage; hence utilize a conduit which quickly achieves this end.
5. *Degree of proximal obstruction.* Common sense dictates that one should not expect a conduit to enhance blood supply to an area if in the native circulation the stenotic area has an internal diameter greater than the lumen of the bypass conduit. This is particularly critical in re-operations where a diseased saphenous vein graft (SVG) may have a stenosis, but the stenotic lumen is equal to or greater than the lumen of an internal thoracic artery (ITA) proposed for bypass to the area. With excision of the diseased SVG, flow via

an ITA in the immediate postoperative period may be less than the myocardium demands and the area will infarct, a catastrophic phenomenon which has been demonstrated many times.
6. *Size and morphology of coronary artery.* As with mismatched size of conduit, there is similar mismatch with size of coronary artery. Not only the size, but the thickness of the artery can be of importance, since a poor anastomosis is likely with an attempt to utilize a small graft to a large, thickened, diseased coronary artery.
7. *Location of anastomosis.* There are limits as to where certain arterial grafts can reach when they are based on their normal inflow. Much of this depends on how much length one can obtain in dissection of the vessel, but also on the position and size of the heart and location of the target coronary artery.
8. *Pathology of the previous grafts and native coronary artery disease.* It is unwise to attempt anastomosis of a small delicate bypass conduit to a large diseased coronary artery. Also, if a previous conduit is severely diseased, regardless of its patency, it should be removed, and hence one needs to select a conduit of equal size.

The ideal vascular graft for any revascularization procedure must exhibit multiple properties, including pliability, easy to handle, resistance to infection, easily procurable, expansible, resistance to arteriosclerosis, inexpensive, incorporates into the body, available in various sizes, unlimited quantity, capable of growth, and have a living endothelial lining. It is obvious that no such graft is presently available and probably will never be available. Some of the grafts exhibit many of the above properties, whereas others exhibit few properties. One should expect that the grafts available at re-operation will be of lesser quality and quantity than those at the primary operation, but this may not be true, depending on what was used initially.

Many types of grafts have been used in coronary bypass grafting, including autogenous veins (greater saphenous, lesser saphenous, and cephalic); autogenous arteries (internal thoracic, splenic, right gastroepiploic, inferior epigastric, and radial); homologous veins (greater saphenous and umbilical); heterogenous arteries (bovine ITA); and prosthetic (PTFE).

SAPHENOUS VEIN

The saphenous vein was the first conduit used as a bypass graft to the coronary arteries. There is no doubt that these veins have been the most common conduit used as of this date. Generally, they are easy to procure and relatively plentiful since there are paired greater and lesser saphenous veins with a total of less than 200 cm in an adult. The long-term patency is variable and unpredictable, although it stands to reason that the technic in harvesting and preparing the vein has some effect on patency. Intimal hyperplasia develops in all veins as the result of *arterization* of the vein and is present within one month after insertion (Figure 1). Fibrous proliferation develops not only on the intima but may also extend into the media. This hyperplasia may develop at such a rapid rate that the vessel may occlude within a month, or it may be a slow reaction, building up only slightly over years.

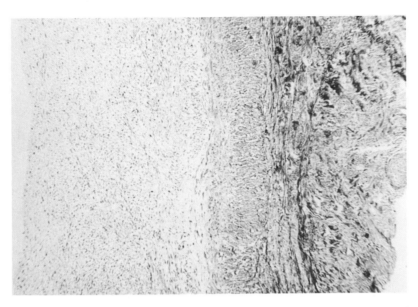

Figure 1. Photomicrograph (125x) of saphenous vein graft shows thick layer of intimal hyperplasia.

By eight years, the majority of saphenous vein grafts have developed arteriosclerotic changes in the intimal hyperplasia, and these changes are also related to the risk factors of the patients. Twenty percent of SVG's develop proximal suture line stenosis and one-fourth of these occlude at five years. Fifty percent of SVG's develop distal suture line stenosis, but the stenosis here does not appear to progress. Ten percent of all saphenous vein grafts close within the first few weeks postoperatively and 50 to 60 percent are closed at ten years. However, the long-term patency of SVG to the left anterior descending artery is relatively high with 80 percent open at ten years.

INTERNAL THORACIC ARTERY

Vascular surgeons, many years ago, demonstrated that autogenous arteries are the best conduit to revascularize any organ, and the heart is no exception. Thus, it is best to select autogenous arteries for revascularization whenever possible and practical.

The internal thoracic artery has been used as a coronary graft for more than 20 years and has demonstrated extremely high patency rates (98 percent at one year and greater than 90 percent at ten years) and rarely closes thereafter.

Many years ago, I asked our pathologists to dissect out both internal thoracic arteries in 25 adult autopsies to determine the histological char-

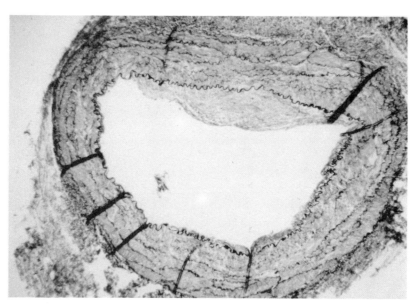

Figure 2. Photomicrograph (50x) of cross section of internal thoracic artery demonstrates small intimal plaque.

acter of the artery. The only lesion we saw among 50 resected specimens was a small intimal plaque which was not hemodynamically significant (Figure 2). To date, we have not seen any internal thoracic artery used as an in situ graft develop intimal hyperplasia or arteriosclerosis postoperatively. While I realize this is a profound and dogmatic statement, it remains unchallenged.

The favorable factors of the ITA are mainly related to the function of the endothelial cells in their production of endothelium-derived relaxing factor and prostaglandin, plus the fact that the media is almost entirely made of elastic tissue. Other favorable factors are that it is an artery of similar size to the coronary arteries to which it is anastomosed; utilized as an in situ graft, it only requires one anastomosis; it has a high velocity flow; it has the ability to grow upon demand; and it is autogenous. On the adverse side, there are only two such arteries and they have a limited length but this is relative since any part of the heart can be reached by one or the other ITA. The most limiting factor is their size; hence, one should not expect an ITA to compete with a native circulation or a previous graft in which the stenotic lumen is larger than the ITA. Another limitation is that only one ITA can be used in diabetic patients because of the inadequate blood supply to the sternum following utilizing both arteries in this condition. As mentioned earlier, the ITA is mainly an elastic artery and less likely to go into spasm than an artery with a highly muscular media. However, it has been demonstrated that the media of the ITA has significant muscle in its proximal portion and also distally as it branches into the musculophrenic and superior epigastric arteries.[1] Therefore, it is wise to utilize this artery significantly proximal to its bifurcation to avoid having an anastomosis with a muscular portion of the artery, and thus avoid spasm.

Selection of Conduits for Primary and Re-Do Operations

Although the ITA has a relatively small diameter, studies have demonstrated that blood flows at normal pressures are negligible if the internal diameter is 2.4 mm or larger. It has been our experience that if one prepares the internal mammary artery properly by hydrostatic dilatation with a diluted blood solution of papaverine, one can always obtain an internal diameter of greater than 2.5 mm. Hence, one should not expect any pressure loss per unit length if the internal diameter is greater than 2.5 mm.[2]

Also, the fact that the internal mammary is narrower than a saphenous vein is not a disadvantage but can be desirable since the velocity of flow is greater, a factor favoring early patency of bypass grafts. It is a known fact that platelets and fibrin deposition on the intimal surface of a graft decreases as the velocity of flow increases. In grafts inordinately larger than the vessel they are bypassing, the fibrin buildup can progress to a point of critical loss in pressure and result in complete thrombotic occlusion.

Flemma et al.[3] demonstrated that flow in the saphenous vein graft was greater than that of an internal mammary artery when connected to the same coronary artery. They anastomosed the internal mammary artery to a saphenous vein graft. We modified this in a clinical experiment by connecting the internal mammary artery and a saphenous vein graft

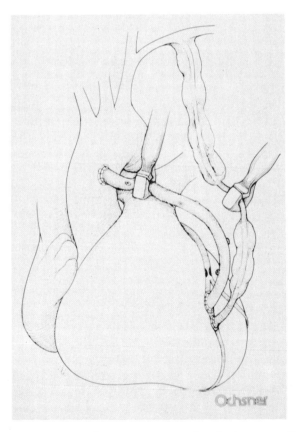

Figure 3. Drawing depicts blood flow measurement by electro-magnetic flowmeter in an internal thoracic artery and saphenous vein graft to the same coronary artery.

separately, but immediately in tandem to the same coronary artery (Figure 3). We corroborated their findings by measuring flow from both the SVG and the ITA at the same time. The flows in the ITA were less than those in the SVG, which one would expect since the flow through the smaller conduit could not compete with the larger conduit. However, when we occlude the SVG, the internal mammary flow increases substantially and approximates that of the SVG.

The ITA can be used in both an in-situ or free graft anastomosed to the aorta. Although a free graft can be more versatile in relation to its length and site of distal anastomosis, it has not demonstrated as high a patency as when used as an in-situ graft.

RIGHT GASTROEPIPLOIC ARTERY

This artery has been a welcome addition to the arterial conduits used to revascularize the heart. The fact that it is an artery allows the intima to secrete vasodilators and also inhibit platelet activity. Although it has an old history in that it was used as far back as 1973,[4] use of the right gastroepiploic (RGE) was discontinued because of an associated high mortality rate. However, in the past five years it has become a popular graft since it has demonstrated a 95 percent patency at five years.[5] Unfortunately, there is only one of these arteries. It is quite cumbersome to work with, in that one needs to ligate each of its branches. The pedicle is very fat and proper alignment is difficult. One needs to procure a fairly lengthy pedicle in order to reach most areas of the heart. Although it can reach many areas of the heart, it is almost exclusively limited to the right coronary artery and its branches. In contrast to the ITA, the RGE has a muscular media and hence is more reactive, and one must take measures to prevent spasm of this vessel. This has fairly well been accomplished by the intra-luminal injection of papaverine and/or verapamil. Like the ITA, the RGE has limited size and flow and should not be used where competitive flow is present. There are no true contraindications to the use of an RGE except a previous operation such as a gastrectomy where it has been sacrificed. Relative contraindications are severe obesity, previous laparotomy or a history of constant abdominal illness.

INFERIOR EPIGASTRIC ARTERY

Use of this artery for myocardial revascularization is fairly new. It has the benefits and limitations of all arteries and yet has not demonstrated the early good patency rate of the internal thoracic and gastroepiploic arteries. The patency of the inferior epigastric artery at six months is 86 percent and, of yet, there are no studies of long-term patency.[6] It does have a limited length, the mean being 12 cm. It can be used only as a free graft, and like the gastroepiploic, has a muscular media with tendencies to spasm.

RADIAL ARTERY

This vessel was used back in the early 70's and its use discontinued in this country after Curtis et al.[7] reported an early patency rate of only 60 percent and a late patency of only 42 percent. However, subsequently Carpentier,[8] who was the first to employ this artery as a bypass graft, demonstrated a 100 percent early patency rate and a 94 percent late patency rate. Carpentier demonstrated that the cause of the poor results was due to spasm of this vessel. He has shown that one needs to take the artery down as a pedicle with its vein and fascia to avoid trauma, to dilate it with dilute papaverine, and to treat the patients at the time of operation and postoperatively with diltiazem hydrochloride to prevent spasm. Others have subsequently begun using this graft again, and in Europe a large experience demonstrates high patency rates.[6] There have been no reports as of this date of loss of hand, since those using this graft have demonstrated the importance of employing the Allen compression test to demonstrate an adequate collateral blood supply to the hand through the ulnar artery. However, because of the litigious nature of our society, many in the United States will be reluctant to use this artery for fear of the severe consequences should an ischemic hand develop.

HOMOLOGOUS VEIN

Homologous saphenous veins have been used as a substitute graft in many areas of the body. However, the results have been varied and not predictable.

Used as a coronary graft, the homologous vein has proved effective. We utilized 38 such grafts as coronary grafts in 31 patients who had insufficient length of autogenous tissue.[9] The homologous vein grafts were used to bypass the least important vessel or vessels. These patients (20 men and 11 women) ranged in age from 43 to 78 years. Fifteen of them reported regular tobacco abuse. Nine were diabetics and 11 had hypertension. The amount of objective followup information on the 38 grafts was limited. There was no operative mortality. In 8 patients, the operation was a repeat operation. Four patients with a total of 7 homologous SVG developed significant recurrent symptoms which necessitated repeat cardiac catheterization. One of these patients had an open homologous graft to the circumflex and right coronary arteries at 15 months postoperatively but died suddenly two years later. No autopsy was performed. In the other three symptomatic patients, there were five homologous grafts, three of which were occluded. Four asymptomatic patients with single homologous graft and multiple autogenous grafts underwent routine angiography at one year. Two homografts were occluded. One was stenotic in the mid portion and the other was widely patent. An additional patient died 19 months postoperative, and autopsy revealed that the homograft to the right coronary artery had recently occluded. Thus, in twelve grafts studied in nine patients (range 1 to 77 mos.), only six were patent.

Homologous veins undergo morphologic changes the minute the graft is removed from the body. The changes show progressive deterioration of the cellular elements. When a homograft vein is placed as an arterial substitute, an early inflammatory reaction occurs with alteration and death of the endothelial cells within a few hours. Degeneration of smooth muscles and fibrous tissue develops less rapidly. There is a gradual fragmentation and eventual disappearance of the elastic tissue. The perivascular fibroblastic reaction and fibroblastic covering of the endothelium lead to progressive narrowing of the lumen. This progressive necrobiosis leads to fibrotic replacement of the graft with varying degrees of cellular life.

In an attempt to lessen the immunologic response of these grafts, cryopreservation and glutaraldehyde fixation have been used. Glutaraldehyde fixation denies the advantages of the handling properties of the homograft; however, it negates the immunologic response. It was hoped that with cryopreservation there would be a greater long-term patency of the homograft; however, this has not proved to be true. Thus, at the present time homologous veins are not a viable option in myocardial revascularization.

HETEROGENOUS BOVINE INTERNAL THORACIC ARTERY

The bovine ITA has many properties which we felt would make it an ideal substitute if it could be treated in such a manner to prevent an immunologic response. Early experience was encouraging;[10] however, it has

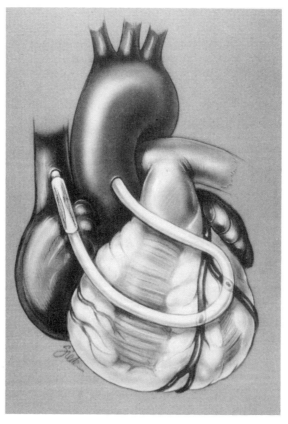

Figure 4. PTFE prosthesis to coronary graft used as an arterial venous fistula with narrowing of lumen proximal to venous anastomosis to produce venturi effect.

been demonstrated that all these grafts occlude with time. Hence, no longer do we consider the bovine ITA as an alternative.

PROSTHETIC GRAFT

Polytetrafluroethylene (PTFE) has been used by us and others as a coronary bypass graft, but early results showed that this graft occluded quite early (Figure 4). The reasons for occlusion are those of any small diameter prosthetic graft where because of the diameter the normal pseudo-intimal lining produces early obstruction. However, recently a new PTFE graft utilizing an arterio-venous fistula with a narrowing of the lumen just proximal to the venous connection allows for continuous flow and yet the venturi effect of the stenosis will allow adequate flow into the coronary arteries and yet continued flow from the arterio-venous fistula. At the present time, this experimental graft is undergoing evaluation and four such grafts have been inserted,[11] which to this day have all remained patent. Thus, this is the first prosthetic graft that has some encouraging results, albeit very early.

DISCUSSION

One needs to individualize for each patient the selection of conduits in myocardial revascularization in both a primary and re-do operation. There is no doubt that many more alternatives are available at a primary operation than a secondary operation. Because certain grafts demonstrate better long-term patency, it behooves all who perform myocardial revascularization to be versed in their use in an attempt to revascularize a heart with little chance for the need of re-operation. On the other hand, one must select the proper conduit or conduits that will not add risk to the patient. Although it has been amply demonstrated that arterial grafts and, in particular, the ITA have superior patency, it stands to reason that in a person with an expected longevity of less than five years, the necessity for using an arterial graft over a saphenous vein is not great. In contrast, in a young man of 60 or under, it is almost imperative that one attempt to perform all revascularization with arterial conduits, particularly those conduits that have demonstrated good long-term patency to this point without question.

It is paramount in a re-operation to avoid using an arterial graft with a small diameter to a coronary artery which is being supplied by a diseased SVG, in which the stenotic area has a larger lumen than the substitute arterial graft. Excision of the SVG will result in immediate decrease in blood supply to the area and a chance for an acute myocardial infarct.

Where there is limited conduit material, one must be cognizant of the benefit of segmental grafting from the same conduit and also of grafting off a parent bypass graft. We have found it particularly useful to use the ITA as a parent graft with a segment of vein or other arterial conduits as saprophyte grafts. However, we believe such measures should be avoided if unnecessary and the ITA (the most proven graft) should be directed to the vessels of greatest importance.

REFERENCES

1. Van Son JAM, et al: Bifurcated ("Y") internal thoracic-coronary artery grafts. J Thorac Cardiovasc Surg 1993;106:945–946.
2. Ochsner JL, Mills NL: Coronary artery surgery. Lea & Febiger, Philadelphia, PA, 1978.
3. Flemma RJ, Singh HM, et al: Comparative hemodynamic properties of veins and mammary artery in coronary bypass operation. Ann Thorac Surg 1975;20:619–627.
4. Edwards WS, Blakely WR, et al: Technique of coronary bypass with autogenous arteries. J Thorac Cardiovasc Surg 1973;65:272–275.
5. Suma H, Wanibushi Y, et al: The right gastroepiploic artery graft: clinical and angiographic: midterm results in 200 patients. J Thorac Cardiovasc Surg 1992;105:615–623.
6. Barner H: Personal communication.
7. Curtis JJ, Stoney WS, et al: Intimal hyperplasia (A cause of radial artery aortocoronary bypass graft failure). Ann Thorac Surg 1975;20:628–635.
8. Acar C, Carpentier A: Revival of the radial artery for coronary artery bypass grafting. Ann Thorac Surg 1992;54:652.
9. Ochsner JL, Lawson JD et al: Homologous veins as an arterial substitute: Long-term results. J Vasc Surg 1984;1:306–313.
10. Suma H, Wanibushi Y, et al: Bovine internal thoracic artery grafts. J Thorac Cardiovasc Surg 1991;32:268.
11. Emery RW, Petersen R, et al: First clinical use of the Possis® synthetic coronary graft. J Cardiovasc Surg 1993;8:439–442.

SURGICAL TREATMENT OF PEDIATRIC AORTIC STENOSIS

Donald B. Doty, M.D.

University of Utah School of Medicine
LDS Hospital
Salt Lake City, Utah

Distortion of the normal anatomy of the aortic root by the processes of congenital malformation presents special problems for the surgeon. Traditionally, obstructions of the left ventricular outflow tract occurring in the aortic root are classified as valvular, subvalvular or supravalvular. There is a spectrum of defects which involve the aortic root with some blending together and overlap of these anomalies.

AORTIC VALVE STENOSIS

Congenital valvular aortic stenosis includes those defects wherein the major malformation involves the aortic valve cusps. There may be an abnormal number of cusps with the valve being described as bicuspid or unicuspid.[1] The most common type of bicuspid valve usually consists of thickened leaflets which arise within a right-left orientation with an anterior and posterior commissure. There is usually a rudimentary raphe or *commissure* in what would be the usual location between right and left coronary cusps. Less common is the two cusp valve with anterior-posterior relationships with the commissures placed on the right and left. The raphe represents the area of commissural fusion between two of three leaflets present in the developing valve. Most bicuspid valves will show three interleaflet triangles on the ventricular side of the cusps indicating that there were three leaflets present in the developing valve. A bicuspid valve with only two definitive leaflets is uncommon and usually not stenotic early in life, rather presenting later in life with obstruction or incompetence of the valve. Occasionally valves will have a tricuspid formation with fusion of the commissures. The size of the valve leaflets are seldom of equal size. This type of valve is most favorable for valvotomy. The so-called *unicuspid or unicommissural valve* has only one posteriorly located commissure which is usually open to the aortic wall. Careful examination of these valves show three sinuses of Valsalva and there are usually three interleaflet triangles on the ventricular side of the valve. The single leaflet valve also appears to be a fusion of three leaflets but it is the least favorable type for valvotomy. The valve cusps are very thickened in all forms of congenital aortic valve stenosis and have dysplastic nodules so that the sheer bulk of the cusps may result in significant obstruction even after the commissures are open. There may be some associated malformation of the structure of the sinus of Valsalva and the entire structure of the aortic root may be small. The left ventricle may also be undersized and there may be associated endocardial fibroelastosis. Early and late prognosis appears to be determined mostly by the size and condition of the left ventricle. Endocardial fibroelastosis is associated with uniformly bad prognosis. According to Leung and associates,[2] small left ventricle (echocardiographic inflow dimension less than 25 mm), small mitral valve orifice (less than 9 mm), and small left ventricle/aortic junction (less than 5 mm) are associated with poor prognosis following aortic valvotomy and patients presenting with size reduction of left heart structures should be considered for hypoplastic left ventricle treatment plans. Gundry and Behrendt[3] also found that endocardial fibroelastosis was predictive of poor outcome but that some infants with critical aortic stenosis benefit from valvotomy even with impaired left ventricular function and severely reduced left ventricular dimensions and may have nearly normal hemodynamics on late follow-up.

Just as there is a spectrum of severity of valvular morphology in patients with congenital aortic valve stenosis, there is a spectrum time and severity of presentation of the condition for treatment. The patients with the worst valve deformity present as neonates with life threatening critical aortic valve stenosis. Less severe forms of valve deformity appear later in childhood with an insidious onset.[4] It is commonly accepted that mild bicuspid malformations of the aortic valve present in adult life as calcareous aortic valve stenosis with the peak occurrence during the fifth decade of life. Vollebergh and Becker[5] suggest that minor inequality of the size of three leaflet valves present from birth may lead to the formation of senile or degenerative type of aortic valve stenosis presenting in the seventh or eighth decade of life. Treatment plans match the presentation of the condition and the age of the patient. The goal of treatment of the critically ill infant is survival and palliative treatment of the valve malformation by aortic valvotomy. For the child, the treatment is elective to preserve left ventricular myocardial function with palliative treatment of the valve by aortic valvotomy whenever this is possible to allow growth to adult size. Aortic valve replacement, however, is occasionally necessary, especially if the valve has become infected. For the adult, elective replacement of the aortic valve is usually recommended to preserve left ventricular performance.

Neonates with critical aortic valve stenosis should have aortic valvotomy soon after adequate resuscitation. Prostaglandin infusion is used to keep the ductus arteriosus open and to generally improve perfusion. The most common method of aortic valvotomy is to perform the procedure on cardiopulmonary bypass usually under direct vision but occasionally as a closed procedure. Using this approach, Turley and associates[6] report 87.5 percent hospital survival in a study which involved three institutions. Most surgeons agree that when the procedure is performed open, the fused commissures are incised to the aortic wall. Rudimentary commissures or raphes are not opened in order to avoid creation of aortic valve incompetence. Ilbawi and associates[7] report use of extended aortic valvuloplasty, in which the commissurotomy incision is extended into the aortic wall around the leaflet insertion, mobilizing the valve cusp attachment at the commissures, and freeing the aortic insertion of the rudimentary commissure. They showed reduced aortic valve gradients compared to standard aortic valvotomy at 1.7 years after operation. Catheter balloon valvotomy is also an acceptable method of opening the aortic valve for relief of critical aortic valve stenosis.[4] The procedure is clearly less invasive than operative aortic valvotomy but also less controlled in terms of what actually happens to the aortic valve. Balloon valvotomy may fail to relieve the obstruction, tear the aortic wall, perforate or avulse an aortic valve leaflet resulting in severe aortic valve incompetence. Nevertheless, in experienced hands, balloon aortic valvotomy may achieve a high rate of successful palliation of aortic valve stenosis. Choice of procedure will depend on individual institutional considerations.

There is considerable data regarding the clinical course of patients having congenital aortic valve stenosis. The Second Natural History Study of Congenital Heart Defects[8] includes data on many patients treated for aortic valvular stenosis and followed for 25 years. The patients analyzed were all two years of age or older at the time of entry into the study. Forty percent of patients managed medically subsequently required surgical management. For patients presenting with left ventricular to aortic pressure gradient greater than 50 mm Hg, 70 percent required surgical intervention. Almost 40 percent of operated patients required a second operation. Three other studies[9-11] which include follow-up data to 20 years or more in patients with congenital aortic valve stenosis over the age of one year treated by aortic valvotomy. These studies show that the risk of the initial operation is low (less than 3.9 percent) but 35–50 percent of them will require a second operation. The rate of reoperation up to ten years is low (2 to 5 percent) and accelerates after that point 3.3 percent per year. Less is known about the long-term results in patients having operations during the neonatal period or at age less than one year. Tveter and associates[10] state that reoperation rate for the newborn-infant group is 5.5 times that for children. Probability or requiring reoperation in neonates less than 28 days old with critical aortic stenosis is 30 percent at the ten year mark for patients having open aortic valvotomy and over 60 percent for those treated by closed technique according to Pelech and associates.[12] It may be possible to perform a second aortic valvotomy for further palliation in these patients. The data from these long-term studies, however, indicates that aortic valve replacement is performed in 74 to 95 percent of second operations. Long-term survival is quite favorable (77 to 85 percent) in patients over one year of age at initial treatment. It should be noted that about one-half of late deaths occur suddenly.[9] Long-term survival data is insufficient for patients having initial treatment in the neonatal period but trends appear to be similar to the older age group after initial hospital mortality is subtracted in spite of the burden of earlier and more frequent reoperation rates.[12]

SUBVALVULAR AORTIC STENOSIS

Subvalvular aortic stenosis includes anomalies causing left ventricular outflow obstruction which are primarily located below the aortic valve. Other anomalies of the heart or great vessels are commonly associated with subaortic stenosis in two-thirds or more of these patients.[15] It is customary to classify the morphology of subvalvular aortic stenosis into two forms: (1) localized membranous or fibromuscular (fixed) form; (2) diffuse or tunnel type. The membranous or fibromuscular form is represented by formation of a discrete fibrous circumferential diaphragm that extends from the septum onto the anterior leaflet of the mitral valve.[1] Patients with the localized form of subaortic stenosis seldom present for treatment before six months of age. Sommerville[13] postulates that the fixed form of subaortic stenosis is an acquired progressive abnormality which is not present at birth. The diffuse or tunnel form is more complex and represents a spectrum of anomalies including fibrous tunnel subaortic stenosis with normal sized aortic valve or hypoplastic aortic root and ranging to include myocardial (muscular) abnormalities of localized hypertrophic obstructive cardiomyopathy (HOCM) or diffuse HOCM. These various types of diffuse subaortic stenosis often blend imperceptibly from one to another expressing some characteristics of the fibrous or muscular forms. There is even some evidence that the fibrous forms of diffuse tunnel subaortic stenosis and hypertrophic obstructive cardiomyopathy may represent anatomical manifestations of the same genetically transmitted disease with different degrees of expression.[1] Vouhe and Neveux[14] make the point that it is not very important from a surgical point of view to make arbitrary differentiation between the various types of diffuse subaortic stenosis because the same surgical problems must be solved in order to relieve obstruction no matter whatever the anatomical nature of the obstacle. They suggest that the perfect delineation of the anatomical features of the left ventricular outflow tract obstruction will provide answers of several important questions. Is the subaortic stenosis localized or diffuse? Is the stenotic segment limited to the subvalvar area, or does it extend to the valvar or supravalvar level? Is the aortic annulus of normal size or hypoplastic? Are the aortic valve cusps normal or abnormal?

Operative intervention to relieve left ventricular outflow tract obstruction usually conforms with signs and symptoms and indications for intervention applied to valvular aortic stenosis. There is evidence, however, that intervention at an earlier age and at a lower left ventricular to aortic gradient (30 mm Hg) may improve late results depending on the extent of relief of obstruction at the initial operation.[15,16] Subaortic stenosis appears to be a progressive disorder and patients who are untreated or who undergo inadequate initial treatment frequently develop increasing obstruction.[4]

Operation is performed on cardiopulmonary bypass using cold cardioplegic arrest of the heart. The localized form of subaortic stenosis is resected by sharp excision, blunt excision as in endarterectomy,[17] or by excision of the membrane plus septal myectomy.[18] The surgical management of diffuse subaortic stenosis best follows the integrated approach proposed by Vouhe and Neveux.[14] This approach seeks two main goals: (1) to obtain complete relief of the left ventricular outflow tract obstruction by the appropriate procedure and (2) to preserve the native aortic valve whenever possible. The approach involves the incisions of the aortoseptal approach, entering the left ventricular outflow tract through the commissure between the right and left aortic valve cusps into the interleaflet triangle and across into the ventricular septum. Each edge of the ventricular septotomy is resected to relieve the subvalvular obstruction. The edges of the septostomy are either closed directly or a patch inserted to further widen the left ventricular outflow tract. The aortic commissure is closed to preserve the normal aortic valve or if the valve is abnormal, it is replaced with a prosthetic valve as part of a complete aortoventriculoplasty (Konno procedure). Clarke[19] has reported use of an aortic allograft root replacement for modified aortoventriculoplasty and Milsom and Doty[20] have used an aortic allograft with attached anterior leaflet of the mitral valve to widen the left ventricular outflow tract posteriorly into the anterior leaflet of the mitral valve for complex localized subvalvular aortic stenosis.

Follow-up studies reveal that there is a significant incidence of reoperation for recurrent or residual subaortic stenosis and for aortic valve incompetence. Stewart and associates[21] found that about one-half of their patients having operations for localized and diffuse forms of subvalvular aortic stenosis required reoperation, some as long as 17 years after the initial procedure. The hazard function for reoperation increased at five years. Lupinetti and associates[22] found that addition of septal myectomy to resection of discrete subaortic stenosis reduced the frequency of reoperation while others[18,23] thought that complete relief of obstruction at the initial operation was more important than whether or not septal myectomy was added to resection of the obstructing membrane. Brown and associates[24] noted association of discrete subvalvular aortic stenosis and aortic valve incompetence and reasoned that early relief of the subaortic obstruction may arrest the progression of the aortic valve lesion. Penoske et al.[15] proposed that operation is indicated if any aortic valve thickening or if even trivial aortic valve incompetence is present, irrespective of the left ventricular to aortic pressure gradient, reasoning that aortic valve incompetence has been shown to be progressive in nature. Rizzoli and associates[16] found mild aortic valve incompetence in 51 and moderate incompetence in 8 of 67 patients operated for discrete subaortic stenosis. Risk factors included older age and higher gradient at time of operation supporting a policy of early repair of discrete subaortic stenosis. Sreeram and associates[25] suggest that intraoperative echocardiography will provide better morphological information about obstructive lesions of the left ventricular outflow tract and enable immediate assessment of the adequacy of operative repair.

SUPRAVALVULAR AORTIC STENOSIS

Supravalvular aortic stenosis is the least common form of left ventricular outflow obstruction. The classification of two forms of the defect is based on what is done from a surgical viewpoint: localized and diffuse types. The localized form encompasses so called *hourglass and membranous forms*. The diffuse form is a condition which involves not only the sinus rim but also the ascending aorta, arch and arch arterial branches. Supravalvular aortic stenosis should be thought of as a complex anomaly of the aortic root.

Too often the surgeon focuses attention on only the defect at the sinus rim. The narrowing and thickening of the sinus rim is fundamental to the morphology of the defect but there is more to understanding this defect. There is thickening of the aortic media and intimal hyperplasia resulting in reduction of the aortic circumference at the sinus rim. The morphologic process may not be circumferential but may only involve the sinus rim over one or two sinuses. The sinus of Valsalva beneath the thick and short sinus rim may be abnormal or hypoplastic. The ostia of the coronary arteries may be obstructed by the overhanging thick sinus rim as well as a bound down aortic cusp. The aortic valve cusps are reported to be thickened in about 30 percent of patients with supravalvular aortic stenosis.[26] The aortic valves are actually involved in every case because the relationships of the commissures are distorted as they are drawn close together by the shortened and thickened sinus rim. This distortion produces a characteristic buckling of the free edge of the aortic valve as the normal length accommodates for the shortened space at the sinus rim. The buckled aortic cusps become part of the obstruction within a space too small to accommodate them properly. The free edge of the aortic cusps usually has normal length in most young patients. Thickening of the edges of the aortic cusps, however, eventually accompanies turbulent blood flow associated with stenosis at the sinus rim. The thickened valve cusps then become an even more important part of the stenosing process. Primary abnormality of the aortic cusps such as bicuspid valve or commissural fusion is often associated with supravalvular aortic stenosis. The edge of the aortic valve cusp may become adherent to the aortic wall isolating the aortic sinus and completely closing the coronary ostia. Subvalvular stenosis of the left ventricular outflow tract may also be part of this total deformity of the aortic root.

Patients with supravalvular aortic stenosis usually present for treatment in childhood when typical ejection type murmur of aortic stenosis is heard. Signs or symptoms of supravalvular stenosis are rarely present in infancy and develop only later during childhood. The natural history is that of progressive left ventricular outflow tract obstruction associated with poor growth of the ascending aorta.[27] Decision for operation is usually based on criteria similar to those for aortic valve stenosis.

Operation to relieve left ventricular outflow tract obstruction caused by the localized form supravalvular aortic stenosis may be accomplished in many cases simply by placing a diamond shaped patch across the sinus rim in the non-coronary sinus of Valsalva. This is the classic operation[28] and will usually reduce or eliminate pressure gradients between the left ventricle and the ascending aorta. Unfortunately, this operation will accomplish little in rebuilding or remodeling the rest of the aortic root abnormalities which usually accompany thickening and narrowing of the sinus rim. It would seem that operations which achieve the best reconstruction of the entire aortic root will have the best chance of giving the patient a better early result and a longer period of time until something more has to be done to the aortic valve or the aortic root. Several years ago we proposed an extended patch aortoplasty in hopes of achieving a more symmetric reconstruction of the aortic root.[29] The sinus rim is divided at two points opposite each other and the incisions extended into both the non-coronary sinus and the right coronary sinus between the right coronary ostium and the commissure between the left and right cusps of the aortic valve. Dividing the sinus rim at two points allows the non-coronary cusp and the right coronary cusp of the aortic valve to stretch out to normal length. The buckling of the valve is relieved as the halves of the aorta are separated anteriorly and posteriorly. The left cusp must also be treated either by resection of the supravalvular thickened rim or by incision into the left sinus of Valsalva to allow anterior displacement of one of the commissures of the valve. This is usually accomplished at the medial commissure but may also be done at the posterior commissure. Once the valve cusps are freed up from entrapment by the supravalvular rim, the aortic sinus may be reconstructed by patch angioplasty. Incisions may even be extended into the ventricular septum or into the anterior leaflet of the mitral valve to relieve accompanying subvalvular obstruction with reconstruction continued to the aortic patch angioplasty. This will provide a symmetric reconstruction of the entire aortic root which, hopefully, will provide the best immediate relief of left ventricular outflow tract obstruction and long preservation of aortic valve function. Brom[30] made incisions into all three aortic sinuses after transection of the aorta and widened the sinus and sinus rim with patches to achieve a symmetric reconstruction of the aortic root. These reconstructive operations are accomplished by insertion of nonflexible prosthetic materials in the aortic root which may not properly support the aortic valve over time. Myers and associates[31] reported a method of V-Y flap in which the thickened and stenosed sinus rim is resected by aortic transection. This method does not employ prosthetic material and may better retain the elastic properties of the aortic root. Chard and Cartmill[32] also completely resected the sinus rim and all thickened stenosing tissues into the sinuses of Valsalva, to the level of the left and right coronary arteries. The ascending aorta is anastomosed primarily to the aortic root after extensive aortic arch mobilization.

Operations to correct the diffuse form of supravalvular aortic stenosis are less well defined. The diffuse form has been treated by a variety of operations including patch aortoplasty, left ventricular apex to aorta conduits, aortic resection with graft replacement, and extensive endarterectomy of the ascending aorta and arch with patch aortoplasty. Sharma and associates[33] reported extensive endarterectomy of the ascending aorta and arch with patch aortoplasty extended to the aortic arch. This approach seems to be a good one because it is directed at the diffuse pathology of the anomaly. Since it is known that the morphologic defect involves the media and intima, it is logical to remove that portion of the aortic wall by endarterectomy. Patch aortoplasty which is short of widening the entire ascending aorta and aortic arch will not correct the aortic obstruction.

Results of treatment of supravalvular aortic stenosis indicate that for the most part pressure gradients from left ventricle to the aorta are relieved by patch angioplasty for the localized form of the defect. Keane and associates[34] showed pressure gradients remaining after operation ranged from 4 to 55 mm Hg with a mean of 27 mm Hg. Pressure gradient remaining intraoperatively following extended patch angioplasty ranged from 0 to 35 mm Hg.[29]

Long-term follow-up data is limited in this unusual anomaly. Sharma and associates[33] reported the total experience with operative treatment of supravalvular aortic stenosis at the Texas Heart Institute. The experience spans a 29 year period and comprises 73 patients, surely the largest single institution experience ever reported. Reason would dictate that significant inferences could be drawn from this vast experience and that the treatment of this condition could be clearly defined. On the contrary, the authors correctly conclude that certain forms of supravalvular aortic stenosis continue to pose a serious challenge to surgical treatment. Perhaps this is because even this large experience placed in perspective only amounts to 2 or 3 cases per year making it difficult to learn from concurrent experience. As the experience accumulates, individual cases are treated individually often based on anecdotal information or recall of most recent experience. There were 24 of 73 patients (32 percent) having isolated, localized form of supravalvular aortic stenosis that were treated by patch aortoplasty. The results were good with only one death occurring in the group (4 percent). Unfortunately, no hemodynamic data is supplied. We can infer that about one-third of the patients in the series had a simple anomaly which could be treated with a simple operation. Patients with a localized form of supravalvular aortic stenosis and some other associated obstructive lesion of the left ventricular outflow tract comprised 33 of the 73 patients (45 percent). These patients required patch aortoplasty plus something else such as aortic valvotomy, aortic valve replacement, or subvalvular resection. From this we learn that about one-half of patients with supravalvular aortic stenosis that are classified as simply localized lesions actually have a complex anomaly of the left ventricular outflow tract. Patients with diffuse form of the defect and those complicated with associated cardiac defects or infection do less well and the results are commensurate with the severity and complexity of the composite of the defects. Late follow-up reveals that 16 of the 73 required a second operation (22 percent) at some time during the follow-up period, and that five patients died late after operation for complex forms of the defect. In our group of 15 patients (unpublished data) followed for ten to twenty years after extended aortoplasty operation, showed that the mean immediate post operative gradient was 20 mm Hg (range 0 to 50 mm Hg) compared to a long-term mean gradient of 32 mm Hg (range 6 to 96 mm Hg). Freedom from reoperation was 69 percent at 11 years. Thus, nearly one-third required a second operation. Univariate analysis revealed that presence of a bicuspid aortic valve was a significant risk factor for reoperation. These data suggest that operations for supravalvular aortic stenosis provide effective long-term relief of the pressure gradient over the sinus rim but the operations are only palliative and many, if not all, patients will eventually require other operations during their life course.

Supravalvular aortic stenosis should be considered as an anomaly which affects the entire aortic root rather than simply one which affects the sinus rim. Operations to correct this defect must be directed at not only widening out the supravalvular aorta but also directed at correcting other lesions in the left ventricular outflow tract.

REFERENCES

1. Maizza AF, Ho SY, Anderson RH: Obstruction of the left ventricular outflow tract: anatomical observations and surgical implications. J Heart Valve Dis 1993;2:66–79.

2. Leung MP, McKay R, Smith A, Anderson RH, Arnold R: Critical aortic stenosis in early infancy: anatomic and echocardiographic substrates of successful open valvotomy. J Thorac Cardiovasc Surg 1991;101:526–35.
3. Gundry SR, Behrendt DM: Prognostic factors in valvotomy for critical aortic stenosis in infancy. J Thorac Cardiovasc Surg 92;747–754.
4. Gaynor JW, Elliott MJ: Congenital left ventricular outflow tract obstruction. J Heart Valve Dis 1992;2:80–93.
5. Vollebergh FEMG, Becker AE: Minor congenital variations of cusp size in tricuspid aortic valves: possible link with isolated aortic stenosis. Br Heart J 1977;39:1006–1011.
6. Turley K, Bove EL, Amato JJ, Iannettoni M, Yeh J, Cotroneo JV, Galdieri RJ: Neonatal aortic stenosis. J Thorac Cardiovasc Surg 1990;99:679–84.
7. Ilbawi MN, DeLeon SY, Wilson WR, Roberson DA, Husayni TS, Quinones JA, Arcilla RA: Extended aortic valvuloplasty: a new approach for the management of congenital valvar aortic stenosis. Ann Thorac Surg 1991;52:663–68.
8. Keane JF, Driscoll DJ, Gersony WM, Hayes CJ, Kidd L, O'Fallon WM, Pieroni DR, Wolfe RR, Weidman SH: Second natural history study of congenital heart defects: results of treatment of patients with aortic valvar stenosis. Circulation 1993;Suppl I(87):I-16–27.
9. Hsieh KS, Keane JF, Nadas AS, Bernhard WF, Castaneda AR: Long-term follow-up of valvotomy before 1968 for congenital aortic stenosis. Amer J Cardiol 1986;85:338–41.
10. Tveter KJ, Foker JE, Moller JH, Ring WS, Lillehei CW, Varco RL: Long-term evaluation of aortic valvotomy for congenital aortic stenosis. Ann Surg 1987;206:496–503.
11. DeBoer DA, Robbins RC, Maron BJ, McIntosh CL, Clark RE: Late results of aortic valvotomy for congenital valvar aortic stenosis. Ann Thorac Surg 1990;50:69–73.
12. Pelech AN, Trusler GA, Olley PM, Rowe RD, Freedon RM: Critical aortic stenosis: survival and management. J Thorac Cardiovasc Surg 1987;94:510–17.
13. Sommerville J: Fixed subaortic stenosis: a frequently misunderstood lesion. Int J Cardiol 1985;8:145–148.
14. Vouhe PR, Neveux JY: Surgical management of diffuse subaortic stenosis: an integrated approach. Ann Thorac Surg 1991;52:654–62.
15. Penkoske PA, Collins-Nakai RL, Duncan NF: Subaortic stenosis in childhood: frequency of associated anomalies and surgical options. J Thorac Cardiovasc Surg 1989;98:852–60.
16. Rizzoli G, Tiso E, Mazzucco A, Daliento L, Rubino M, Tursi V, Fracasso A: Discrete subaortic stenosis: operative age and gradient as predictors of late aortic valve incompetence. J Thorac Cardiovasc Surg 1993;106:95–104.
17. McKay R, Ross DN: Technique for the relief of discrete subaortic stenosis. J Thorac Cardiovasc Surg 1982;84:917–20.
18. Cain T, Campbell D, Paton B, Clarke D: Operation for discrete subvalvular aortic stenosis. J Thorac Cardiovasc Surg 1984;87:366–70.
19. Clarke DR: Extended aortic root replacement with cryopreserved allografts: do they hold up? Ann Thorac Surg 1991;52:669–73.
20. Milsom FP, Doty DB: Aortic valve replacement and mitral valve repair with allograft. J Cardiac Surg 1993;8:350–57.
21. Stewart JR, Merrill WH, Hammon JW Jr, Graham TP, Bender HW: Reappraisal of localized resection for subvalvar aortic stenosis. Ann Thorac Surg 1990;50:197–203.
22. Lupinetti FM, Pridjian AK, Callow LB, Crowley DC, Beekman RH, Bove EL: Optimum treatment of discrete subaortic stenosis. Ann Thorac Surg 1992;54:467–71.
23. Ashraf H, Cotroneo J, Dhar N, Gingell R, Roland M. Dieroni D, Subramanian S: Long-term results after excision of fixed subaortic stenosis. J Thorac Cardiovasc Surg 1985;90:864–71.
24. Brown J, Stevens L, Lynch L, Caldwell R, Girod D, Hurwitz R, Mahony L, King H: Surgery for discrete subvalvular aortic stenosis; actuarial survival, hemodynamic results, and acquired aortic regurgitation. Ann Thorac Surg 1985;2:151–155.
25. Sreeram N, Sutherland GR, Bogers AJJC, Stumper O, Hess J, Bos E, Quaegebeur JM: Subaortic obstruction: intraoperative echocardiography as an adjunct to operation. Ann Thorac Surg 1990;50:579–85.
26. Williams JCP, Barratt-Boyes BG, Lowe JB: Supravalvular aortic stenosis. Circulation 1961;24:1311.

27. Wren C, Oslizlok P, Bull C: Natural history of supravalvar aortic stenosis and pulmonary artery stenosis. J Am Coll Cardiol 1990;15:1631–32.
28. McGoon DC, Mankin HT, Vlad P, Kirklin JW: Surgical treatment of supravalvular aortic stenosis. J Thorac Cardiovasc Surg 1961;41:125–133.
29. Doty DB, Polansky DB, Jenson CB: Supravalvular aortic stenosis. J Thorac Cardiovasc Surg 1977;74:362–371.
30. Brom AG: Obstruction to the left ventricular outflow tract. In Khonsari S, (ed) Cardiac surgery: safeguards and pitfalls in operative technique. Rockville, MD: Aspen, CO, 1988;276–80.
31. Myers JL, Waldhausen JA, Cyran SE, Gleason MM, Weber HS, Baylen BG: Results of surgical repair of congenital supravalvular aortic stenosis. J Thorac Cardiovasc Surg 1993;105:281–288.
32. Chard RB, Cartmill TB: Localized supravalvar aortic stenosis: a new technique for repair. Ann Thorac Surg 1993;782–84.
33. Sharma BK, Fujiwara H, Hallman GL, Ott DA, Reul GJ, Cooley DA: Supravalvar aortic stenosis: a 29-year review of surgical experience. Ann Thor Surg 1991;51:1031–39.
34. Keane JF, Fellows KE, LaFarge CG, Nadas AS, Bernhard WF: The surgical management of discrete and diffuse supravalvar aortic stenosis. Circulation 1976;54:112–17.1

SURGICAL AND BIOENGINEERING ADVANCES IN THE TREATMENT OF LIFE THREATENING VENTRICULAR ARRHYTHMIAS

Alden H. Harken, M.D., Patricia A. Kelly, M.D.,
David Mann, M.D., Roger S. Damle, M.D.,
and Michael Reiter, M.D.

University of Colorado
Denver, Colorado

The marriage of bioengineering, electrophysiology and surgery has created gratifying progress in the therapeutic control of cardiac electrical activation. In April of 1930, Albert Hyman received a grant to develop an *artificial pacemaker*. Two years later he successfully paced a human heart with a needle electrode for eight minutes.[1] Two decades later, Seymour Furman successfully established chronic ventricular pacing via transthoracic leads and a *semiambulatory power source* (Figure 1).

By 1960, William Chardack, in collaboration with Andrew A. Gage and an electrical engineer, William Greatbatch, collaborated to produce and place the first successful implantable cardiac pacemaker (Figure 2).

Remarkably it is now possible to place a biphasic tiered-therapy implantable cardioverter/defibrillator without a thoracotomy and with approximately the same magnitude left subcostal bulge. Early fixed rate ventricular pacing could not be temporally related to the spontaneous electrical activity of the heart and was therefore the forerunner of our current electrophysiologic studies (EPS). It was soon learned that exogenous electrical stimuli, while life-saving for bradyarrhythmias, might be life-threatening during tachyarrhythmias. Programmed electrical stimulation permits the introduction of precisely timed impulses that span electrical diastole (Figure 3).

Inducible ventricular tachyarrhythmias by programmed stimulation are defined as *reentrant* while noninducible rhythm disorders are perceived as *automatic*. This apparently trivial electrophysiologic discrimination has enormous therapeutic import.[2] The purposes of this chapter are:

Cardiac Surgery: Current Issues 3, Edited by A. C. Cernaianu and A. J. DelRossi,
Plenum Press, New York, 1995

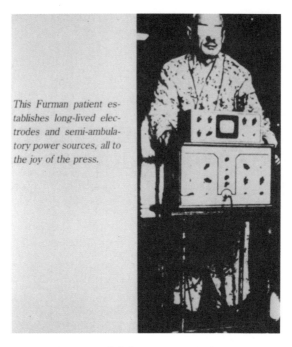

Figure 1. Seymour Furman's successful chronic ventricular pacing via transthoracic leads.

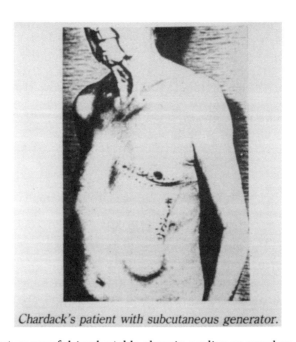

Figure 2. The first successful implantable chronic cardiac pacemaker. Note the anterior thoracotomy scar for placement of epicardial leads and the subcostal bulge comparable to a current AICD.

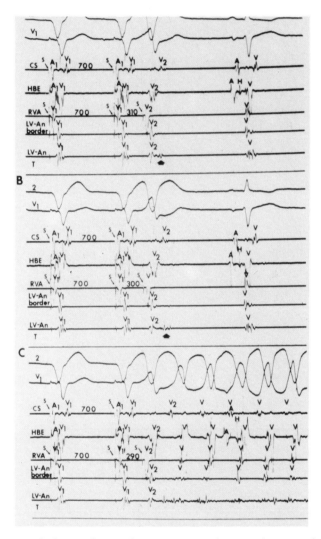

Figure 3. Programmed electrical stimulation permits the introduction of precisely timed impulses that span electrical diastole. Seven concurrent electrograms are presented. Lead II (II), Lead V₁ (VI), coronary sinus (CS), HIS bundle electrogram (HBE), right ventricular anterior wall (RVA), left ventricular aneurysm border (LV-An border) and left ventricular aneurysm (LV-An), trained stimuli (S) are provided at a 700 msec cycle length followed by a single extrasystole at 310msec (panel A). In panel B, the identical train is followed by an extra stimulus of 300 msec, again capturing the ventricle but not sustaining ventricular tachycardia. In panel C, the single extra stimulus at 290 msec enters the reentrant electroanatomic circuit provoking sustained ventricular tachycardia.

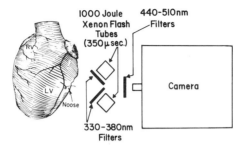

Figure 4. An isolated crystalloid perfused rat heart is maintained on a modified Langendorff apparatus. Excitatory light energy is provided through filters by two 1000 J Xenon flash tubes. NADH fluoresces at 470 nm depicting the area of anoxic myocardium subtended by the noose occlusion of the coronary artery.

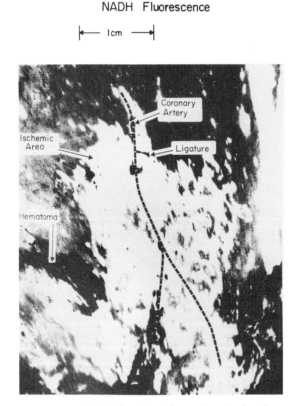

Figure 5. The coronary artery of a dog has been ligated, and after five minutes of ischemia, the myocardium is excised and quick frozen in liquid nitrogen. Dark areas are well perfused oxygenated myocardium. The light area distal to the coronary artery ligature is anoxic identified by reduced NADH. Note the luxuriant coronary arterial collaterals in the dog studded with islands of pericollateral oxygenated and healthy myocardium. This heterogenous ischemic zone is formidably arrhythmogenic.

1. To describe the electroanatomy of ventricular tachyarrhythmias;
2. To explore current indications and experience with electrophysiologically directed endocardial excision for ventricular tachycardia;
3. To examine the currently available implantable automatic defibrillator/cardioverter devices; and
4. To develop an algorithm for the appropriate therapy of patients who present with life-threatening ventricular tachyarrhythmias.

ELECTROANATOMY OF VENTRICULAR ARRHYTHMIAS

The mechanism of ventricular tachycardia is enhanced automaticity, reentry or a combination of both.[3] Automatic ventricular tachycardia is common in the perioperative and peri-infarction periods. Reentrant ventricular tachycardia is most frequently associated with chronic ischemic heart disease. An anatomically heterogeneous ischemic zone of myocardium permits an impulse to enter a stippled area and exit sufficiently late that it may *reenter* the circuit over and over again providing the substrate for reentrant ventricular tachycardia.[2,3] The natural fluorescence of nicotinamide adenine dinucleotide (NADH) permits the photographic display of myocardial zones that are ischemic versus zones that are well perfused[4-6] (Figure 4).

When the epicardial surface of a perfused heart is energized with 370 nm light, resident NADH (ischemic myocardium) naturally fluoresces. This fluorescent NADH emits at a wave length of 470 nm and can be documented on photographic film. When the coronary artery of a dog is ligated, the subtended myocardium develops a heterogeneously ischemic pattern (Figure 5).

Note that the luxuriant coronary arterial collaterals in a dog produce a myocardial infarction zone that is studded with islands of pericollateral healthy myocardium. For this reason, the heterogenous myocardial infarction in a dog is highly arrhythmogenic, while the homogeneous infarct zone in the rabbit, pig and monkey is not.[7] Interestingly, the structure and ultrastructure of subendocardial regions in which ventricular tachycardia originates in human specimens confirms this microanatomical model.[8]

SURGICAL ENDOCARDIAL RESECTION FOR MALIGNANT VENTRICULAR TACHYCARDIA

Epicardial and endocardial electrophysiologic mapping of patients in ventricular tachycardia permitted the identification of the *earliest* site of ventricular activation.[9,10] Our initial premise was that the origin of ventricular tachycardia could be electrophysiologically identified, and its excision would eliminate resultant malignant ventricular arrhythmia.[9,10] Comparison of standard aneurysmectomy against aneurysmectomy with endocardial resection for treatment of recurrent sustained ventricular tachycardia indicated that the electrophysiologically directed surgical approach was both safer and more effective.[11]

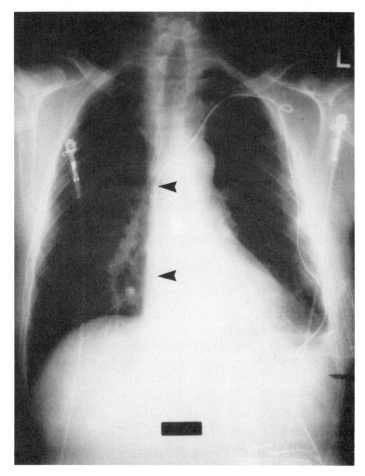

Figure 6. A chest x-ray of a patient following implantation of an AICD with an intracardiac electrode/subcutaneous patch system. The arrows indicate the limits of the intravascular electrode placed at the right atrial/superior vena caval junction. Note the left anterior chest wall subcutaneous patch.

IMPLANTABLE CARDIOVERTER DEFIBRILLATORS

The development of implantable cardioverter defibrillator (ICD) has offered an innovative bioengineering answer to life threatening ventricular arrhythmias.[12-15] The recognition and introduction of defibrillators with biphasic wave forms has permitted successful implantable cardioversion with lower energy systems.[16,17] The delivery of a biphasic truncated exponential wave form has proved effective in clinical cardioversion of ventricular tachycardia/fibrillation in man.[18] Recently, we have reported[19] our experience with 38 patients in whom we implanted a biphasic device (Ventritex® Cadence tiered therapy defibrillator system, Ventritex, Inc., Sunnyvale, CA) utilizing a nonthoracotomy lead system. We have compared this experience with our previous patient population in whom implantable cardioversion was accomplished with an intracardiac lead and a left anterior thoracic subcutaneous patch electrode (Figure 6).

In a period of ten months ending in August of 1993, thirty-eight patients underwent implantation of a Ventritex® Cadence tiered therapy defibrillatory system using a nonthoracotomy approach. In two of the 38 patients, the defibrillation threshold using this configuration was unacceptably high and a thoracotomy was performed. Electrophysiologic studies were performed preoperatively in 37 of the 38 patients. All but one of the patients with inducible ventricular tachycardia underwent antiarrhythmic drug testing. Four patients remained on antiarrhythmic drugs at the time of device implantation. These drugs were necessary for control of frequent episodes of ventricular tachycardia in three patients, or atrial fibrillation in one patient. In all other patients, antiarrhythmic medications were discontinued at least five half lives prior to surgery.

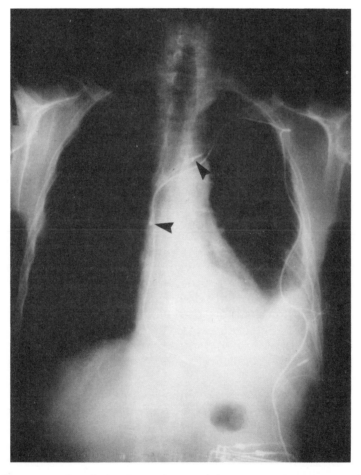

Figure 7. The patient identified in Figure 6 now exhibits proximal migration and dislocation of the intracardiac electrode (arrows). Note that this proximal migration has occurred despite a redundant loop of electrode secured with multiple sutures in the subclavicular prepectoral area.

ICD DEVICE IMPLANTATION

Under general anesthesia, all patients were monitored with an indwelling arterial and pulmonary artery catheters. We have since stopped using pulmonary artery catheters routinely. Under fluoroscopic guidance, a bipolar tined endocardial lead (Cardiac Pacemakers, St. Paul, Minnesota, Model No. BT10) was positioned in the right ventricular apex via the subclavian vein. Once adequate sensing and pacing thresholds were obtained, the lead was anchored in place using several tacking stitches and coiling the electrode in the prepectoral space (in the subclavian prepectoral space) (Figure 6). Once adequate and sensing thresholds were obtained, a coil electrode was positioned at the high right atrial superior vena caval junction using the same subclavian vein. A large patch (Cardiac Pacemakers, Inc., Model L67) was placed subcutaneously near the cardiac apex (Figure 6). Intraoperative testing was performed using a programmable stimulator/cardioverter/defibrillator pacing analyzer (Ventritex, Inc. Model HVS-02). A synchronized biphasic shock of 400 to 600 v was delivered in sinus rhythm in order to determine the impedance of the defibrillating leads. The pulse width of the cardioverting shock was then adjusted according to the measured impedance. Ventricular fibrillation was then induced by rapid ventricular pacing. A synchronized biphasic shock of 600 v was delivered during fibrillation. If the initial 600 v shock was successful, the energy was decreased to 500 v and the process repeated. Further trials were performed as necessary until a minimum of two successful cardioversions was accomplished. This voltage was defined as the defibrillation threshold.

Of the 38 nonthoracotomy implantations we attempted, thirty-six were completed with adequate defibrillation thresholds. The impedance between the coil and the patch during measurement of defibrillation threshold ranged from 31 to 77 ohms. We experienced no perioperative mortality. One patient developed a pneumothorax and one a hemopneumothorax after left subclavian vein puncture. Both required a chest tube only. One patient with chronic atrial fibrillation who converted to sinus rhythm during defibrillation threshold testing, required emergent aortic embolectomy for a saddle embolus (presumably derived from the left atrium during EPS testing) to the aortic bifurcation several hours postoperatively. In this same patient, a chest roentgenogram performed four days following implantation revealed migration of the cardioverting lead (Figure 7).

Thirty-six patients have been followed for a median of 22 weeks. None have died during the follow-up period. Fifteen patients (42 percent) have experienced 53 device discharges. Review of the 42 available stored electrograms from these events suggest that discharges were precipitated by ventricular tachycardia/fibrillation in 12 patients, atrial fibrillation in four patients and sinus tachycardia in two patients. Eight patients had 24 aborted shocks. Spurious discharges for sinus tachycardia or atrial fibrillation occurred in six patients (17 percent) and were clearly diagnosed by the stored electrograms.[19]

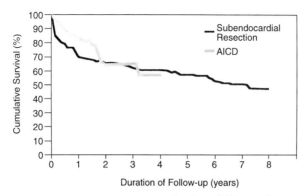

Figure 8. It is perhaps silly to compare survival when different therapies are applied to different patient cohorts. The temptation however is overwhelming. Cumulative survival appears similar following curative subendocardial resection (including peri-operative mortality) for recurrent sustained medically refractory ventricular tachycardia versus implantation (including peri-operative mortality) of an intracardiac cardioverter defibrillator (AICD).

COMPLEMENTARY ICD WITH DEFINITIVE SURGICAL RESECTION FOR MALIGNANT VENTRICULAR TACHYARRHYTHMIAS

When confronted with a patient who has suffered a frightening episode of ventricular tachycardia/fibrillation (*sudden cardiac death*), the physician must first sort out the therapeutic options. The low morbidity and mortality of the currently available ICD devices has great appeal. It is perhaps inappropriate to compare survival when different therapy is applied to different patient cohorts. The temptation, however, is overwhelming (Figure 8).

It appears that curative surgical resection (including perioperative mortality) enjoys an essentially identical cumulative survival with an implanted cardioverter defibrillator (again including perioperative mortality). Moreover, it is perhaps appropriate to stress that the patients presenting predominantly with ventricular fibrillation, and therefore, treated with an ICD may never again exhibit ventricular tachyarrhythmias, while the surgically treated group must have medically refractory inducible recurrent sustained ventricular tachycardia. Thus the groups are truly *not* comparable; the cumulative survival however *is*. As anticipated, electrophysiologically directed surgical therapy is typically curative.[12,13,15] While an implantable cardioverter defibrillator effectively rescues patients with malignant ventricular tachyarrhythmias, it is not designed to prevent these cardiac rhythm disorders. Thus, the *arrhythmia free survival* following implantation of an intracardiac cardioverter defibrillator is approximately 30 percent at four years while *arrhythmia free survival* following corrective endocardial resection approaches 90 percent (Figure 9).

The initial discrete *dichotomy* in the diagnostic/therapeutic road is to determine whether the patient has inducible ventricular tachycardia by programmed stimulation. If ventricular fibrillation or *unmappable* polymor-

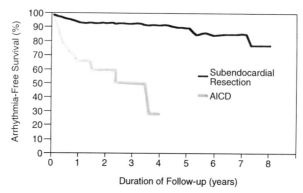

Figure 9. An implantable cardioverter defibrillator effectively rescues patients with malignant ventricular tachyarrhythmias, it is not designed to prevent these cardiac rhythm disorders. Thus, the *arrhythmia free survival* following implantation of an intracardiac cardioverter defibrillator is approximately 30 percent at four years, while *arrhythmia free survival* following corrective endocardial resection approaches 90 percent.

phic ventricular tachyarrhythmias are exclusively inducible, then the only available surgical therapy is an implantable device.

ALGORITHM FOR THE THERAPY OF VENTRICULAR TACHYCARDIA

If the patient presents with hemodynamically stable or hemodynamically unstable ventricular tachycardia, surgical and bioengineering options are available (Figure 10). Pivotal to this early evaluation is a determination of the patients interest in employment and the patient's desire to drive an automobile. An ICD precludes the patient's ability to obtain a driver's license. Again, although the groups are not comparable, patients following

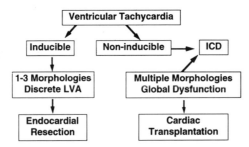

Figure 10. The therapeutic algorithm for ventricular tachycardia hinges on the inducible and therefore mappable nature of this cardiac rhythm. If the rhythm is not inducible, and the patient has tolerable ventricular function, an intracardiac cardioverter defibrillator is appropriate. Patients with electrically unstable severe cardiac dysfunction may be candidates for cardiac transplantation. If a patient has inducible and therefore mappable morphologies of ventricular tachycardia and a discrete left ventricular aneurysm, they may be offered curative endocardial resection.

curative surgical endocardial resection seem more likely physically and psychologically to return to full employment.

If the initial electrophysiologic study indicates sustained, inducible ventricular tachycardia, then we attempt to *map* this rhythm. If the patient presents with more than one morphology of ventricular tachycardia, we make an attempt to locate the origin of each pattern of ventricular tachycardia acknowledging that many morphologies have the same origin and seem to *exit* along divergent pathways. We also catheterize these patients to assess the status of their coronary arteries and to examine their ventricular dysfunction. Approximately two-thirds of patients exhibit concurrent *operable* coronary artery disease. A discrete anterior left ventricular aneurysm is a finding favorable to surgical correction. An inferior aneurysm is also surgically amendable, however, endocardial mapping and excision is somewhat more difficult and the success rate is lower.[14] Thus, the fewer the number of ventricular tachycardia morphologies, and the more discrete the left ventricular aneurysm, the more favorable candidate the patient is for electrophysiologically directed endocardial resection. With increasing number of ventricular tachycardia morphologies and with increasing *global* left ventricular dysfunction, the patient is more likely to be a candidate for an ICD. In patients with severely limiting left ventricular dysfunction and concomitant ventricular tachycardia/fibrillation, we have proceeded with cardiac transplantation, with or without an intervening ICD. Ultimately, the decision concerning therapeutic approach incorporates the patient's interest in employment, interest in driving an automobile, inducibility of ventricular tachycardia/fibrillation, antiarrhythmic pharmacologic suppression of ventricular tachyarrhythmias, concurrent disease, global left ventricular dysfunction and the discreet nature of a left ventricular aneurysm.[20]

During the past fifteen years, electrophysiologists, bioengineers, and surgeons have collaborated on developing a variety of therapeutic options for malignant ventricular tachyarrhythmias that typically complement each other in offering patients gratifyingly successful therapy.

REFERENCES

1. Harken DE: Pacemakers, past-makers and the paced: an informal history from A to Z (Aldini to Zoll). Biomedical Instrumentation and Technology 1991;25:299–321.
2. Harken AH: Surgical treatment of cardiac arrhythmias. Scientific American 1993;269;68–74.
3. Harken AH, Horowitz LN, Josephson ME: The surgical treatment of ventricular tachycardia. Ann Thor Surg 1980;30(5):499–508.
4. Harken AH, Barlow CH, Chance B: Evaluation of myocardial oxygen supply-demand by NADH fluorescence photography. Surg Forum 1977;28:270–272.
5. Harden WR, Simson MB, Barlow CH, Soriano R, Harken AH: Display of epicardial ischemia by reduced nicotinamide adenine dinucleotide fluorescence photography, electron microscopy and ST segment mapping. Surgery 1978;83(6):732–740.
6. Harken AH, Barlow CH, Harden WR, Chance B: Two and three dimensional display of myocardial ischemic "border zone" in dogs. Am J Cardiol 1978;42:954–959.
7. Harken AH, Simson MB, Haselgrove J, Wetstein L, Harden WR, Barlow CH: Early ischemia after complete coronary ligation in the rabbit, dog, pig, and monkey. Am J Physiol 1981;241:H202-H210.

8. Fenoglio Jr JJ, Pham TD, Harken AH, Horowitz LN, Josephson ME, Wit AL: Recurrent sustained ventricular tachycardia: structure and ultrastructure of subendocardial regions in which tachycardia originates. Circulation 1983;68(3):518–533.
9. Harken AH, Josephson ME, Horowitz LN: Surgical endocardial resection for the treatment of malignant ventricular tachycardia. Ann Surg 1979;190:456–460.
10. Horowitz LN, Harken AH, Kastor J, Josephson ME: Ventricular resection guided by epicardial and endocardial mapping for the treatment of recurrent ventricular tachycardia. N Engl J Med 1980;302:589–593.
11. Harken AH, Horowitz LN, Josephson ME: Comparison of standard aneurysmectomy and aneurysmectomy with endocardial resection for the treatment of recurrent sustained ventricular tachycardia. J Thorac Cardiovasc Surg 1980;80:527–534.
12. Mirowski M, Reid PR, Winkle RA: Mortality in patients with implanted automatic defibrillators. Ann Intern Med 1983;98:585–588.
13. Echt DS, Armstrong K, Schmidt P, Oyer P, Stinson E, Winkle RA: Clinical experience, complications and survival in 70 patients with the automatic implantable cardioverter/defibrillator. Circulation 1985;71:289–296.
14. Marchlinski FE, Flores BT, Buxton AE: The automatic implantable cardioverter-defibrillator: Efficacy, complications and device failures. Ann Intern Med 1986;104:481–488.
15. Kelly PA, Cannom DS, Garan H: The automatic implantable cardioverter-defibrillator: Efficacy, complications and survival in patients with malignant ventricular arrhythmias. J Am Coll Cardiol 1988;11:1278–1286.
16. Fromer M, Schlapfer J, Fischer A, Kappenberger L: Experience with a new implantable pacer-cardioverter-defibrillator for the therapy of recurrent sustained ventricular tachyarrhythmias: a step toward a universal ventricular tachyarrhythmia control device. PACE 1991;14:1288–1298.
17. Klein LS, Miles WM, Zipes DP: Antitachycardia devices: realities and promises. J Am Coll Cardiol 1991;18:1349–1362.
18. Winkle RA, Mead RH, Ruder MA: Improved low energy defibrillation efficacy in man with the use of a biphasic truncated exponential waveform. Am Heart J 1989;177:122–127.
19. Kelly PA, Mann DE, Harken AH, Manart FD, Reiter MJ: Implantation of an automatic defibrillator using a simplified nonthoracotomy approach. Submitted for publication, Circulation 1993.
20. Miller JM, Kienzle MG, Harken AH, Josephson ME: Subendocardial resection for ventricular tachycardia: predictors of surgical success. Circulation 1984;70(4):624–631.

LESS HEPARIN FOR CARDIOPULMONARY BYPASS

Ludwig K. von Segesser, M.D., Branko M. Weiss, M.D.*,
Michele Genoni, M.D., Boris Leskosek, and
Marko I. Turina, M.D.

Clinic for Cardiovascular Surgery
and *Institute for Anesthesiology
University Hospital
Zurich, Switzerland

INTRODUCTION

Following the discovery of heparin at the beginning of this century by McLean,[1] cardiopulmonary bypass was introduced into clinical practice in 1952 by John Gibbon.[2] At that time, very complex perfusion equipment was used and cardiopulmonary bypass was a cumbersome procedure. Substantial progress has been made since. Development of disposable oxygenators with improved handling, reduction of priming volume allowing for perfusion without blood prime, and the introduction of membranous gas/blood interfaces with predictable gas transfer rates were some of the main steps in this evolution. Soon after its introduction, the pump oxygenator was also used for distal perfusion during surgery of the descending thoracic aorta. Severe bleeding complications were the major drawback of this approach as long as full systemic heparinization was necessary during perfusion of these patients with very large surgical exposures. Heparin surface bonding in order to reduce the thrombogenicity of artificial surfaces was initiated by V. Gott in 1963[3] who also reported clinical application of heparinized shunts for thoracic aortic surgery without full systemic heparinization.[4] The somewhat limited blood flow of passive apico-aortic shunting triggered further research.

EXPERIMENTAL LEFT HEART BYPASS WITH HEPARIN COATED EQUIPMENT

In a first step, we used a roller pump to increase shunt flow in the experimental set-up. For this purpose, two TDMAC heparin coated shunts

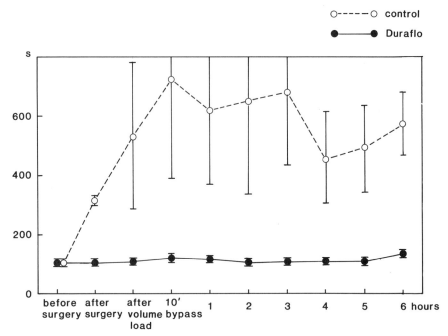

Figure 1. Activated coagulation time (mean ± standard deviations) for perfusion using heparin coated equipment without systemic heparinization as compared to uncoated

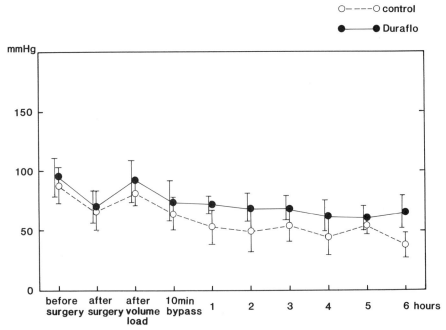

Figure 2. Mean arterial blood pressure (mean ± standard deviations) for perfusion using heparin coated equipment without systemic heparinization as compared to uncoated equipment with full systemic heparinization (control).

(Sherwood Medical, St. Louis, MO, USA) were connected with an electromagnetic flow probe and left heart bypass (left atrium to aorta) was realized in canine experiments. Superior shunt flows without systemic heparinization were realized in this fashion (von Segesser et al., unpublished data). However, the lack of suitable connectors with improved thromboresistance prevented clinical application at that time.

A more complex left heart bypass system was studied after introduction of Duraflo heparin surface coating.[5] Heparin coated tubing sets including cannulas, connectors, tubings and pump loops (Baxter-Bentley, Irvine, CA, USA) were evaluated in canine experiments. For this purpose, an inlet-pressure servo-controlled roller pump (modified Stöckert pump, Munich, Germany) was used. Two groups of animals were perfused over 6 hours using either heparin coated tubing sets without systemic heparinization or uncoated tubing sets with full systemic heparinization. Similar to clinical practice, full systemic heparinization was defined as activated coagulation time (ACT) greater than 480 sec. ACT levels for the two analyzed groups are shown in Figure 1.

In accordance to the protocol, the values measured for the coated group remained within the normal range whereas they were significantly higher for the control group. At the end of the perfusion period, the mean aortic pressure was significantly higher in the group perfused with coated equipment as compared to uncoated controls (Figure 2).

Mixed venous oxygen saturation was again superior in the group perfused with coated equipment as compared to uncoated controls where values below 50 percent were observed (Figure 3).

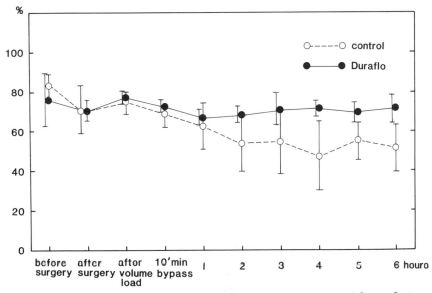

Figure 3. Mixed venous oxygen saturation (mean ± standard deviations) for perfusion using heparin coated equipment without systemic heparinization as compared to uncoated equipment with full systemic heparinization (control).

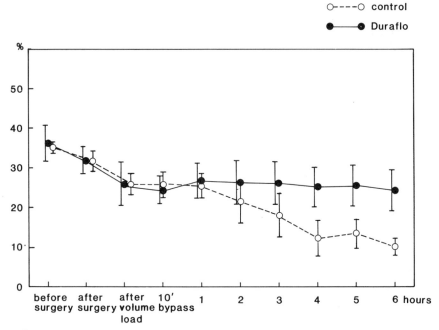

Figure 4. Hematocrit (mean ± standard deviations) for perfusion using heparin coated equipment without systemic heparinization as compared to uncoated equipment with full systemic heparinization (control).

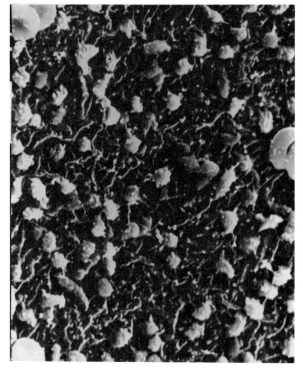

Figure 5. Scanning electron microscopic view of uncoated control surface perfused with full systemic heparinization (ACT>480 sec) over 10 minutes (original magnification 1000x).

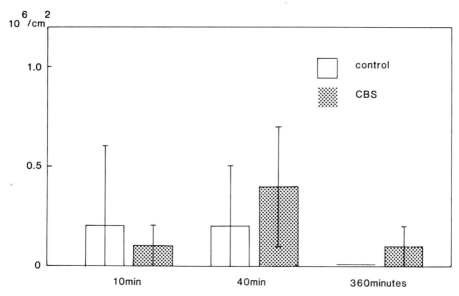

Figure 6. Morphometric analyses: red cell densities on heparin coated surfaces (CBS) perfused without systemic heparinization and uncoated control surfaces perfused with full systemic heparinization (mean±standard deviation: NS).

These differences can be explained by the decreasing hematocrit levels in the group perfused with uncoated equipment (Figure 4) which is due to significantly higher blood loss as a result of full systemic heparinization. After weaning from left heart bypass, macro- and microscopic analyses showed similar amounts of deposits on heparin coated surfaces perfused without systemic heparinization[6] as compared to uncoated surfaces perfused with full systemic heparinization. Interestingly, perfusion without systemic heparin resulted not only in reduced blood loss and transfusion requirements but also in improved renal function and attenuated hormonal responses.[7]

A different approach for heparin surface coating was reported by Larm et al.[8] For evaluation of this coating, we realized a left heart bypass study[9] in canine experiments using CBAS heparin coated components (Carmeda, Stockholm, Sweden) as reported above. After 6 hours of perfusion, blood loss totaled 0.3±0.1 L for heparin coated equipment without systemic heparinization as compared to 1.3±0.5 L for standard equipment with full systemic heparinization ($p<0.01$). Transfusion requirements were 1.1±0.7 L for coated equipment without systemic heparinization as compared to 2.5±0.8 L for uncoated equipment with full systemic heparinization ($p<0.01$). Urine output was significantly higher for coated equipment without systemic heparinization as compared to uncoated with full systemic heparinization (0.9±0.3 L vs. 0.5±0.2 L, $p<0.05$). Blood exposed surfaces of both groups were analyzed with a scanning electron microscope before bypass, 10 minutes after onset of perfusion, as well as after 45 minutes and after 360 minutes of bypass.[10] The scanning electron micrographic pictures were morphometrically analyzed after final photographic magnification

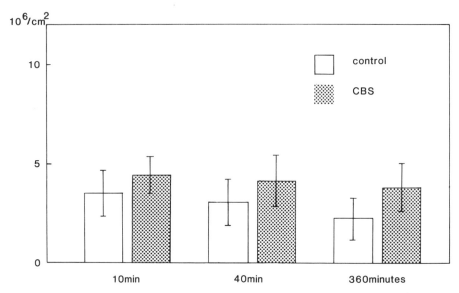

Figure 7. Morphometric analyses: platelet densities on heparin coated surfaces (CBS) perfused without systemic heparinization and uncoated control surfaces perfused with full systemic heparinization (mean±standard deviation: NS).

(magnification x 1000). More than 150 fields were analyzed per surface, timepoint, and animal studied. Overall appearance of heparin coated surfaces exposed to blood without systemic heparinization was similar to that of uncoated control surfaces with full systemic heparinization (Figure 5).

The absolute densities of red cells and platelets are shown in Figures 6 and 7 respectively. There is no significant difference between the two analyzed groups.

In a next step, centrifugal pump heads (Biomedicus®, Minneapolis, MN, USA) were heparin coated (CBAS; Carmeda, Stockholm, Sweden) and evaluated in a bovine left heart bypass model. Again, heparin coated equipment was studied without systemic heparinization and compared to uncoated equipment with full systemic heparinization.[11] As for roller pump left heart bypass without systemic heparinization, reduced blood loss and superior hemodynamics resulted for centrifugal pump left heart bypass using heparin coated equipment without systemic heparinization. Furthermore, the heparin coated pump heads remained macroscopically clean.

EXPERIMENTAL CARDIOPULMONARY BYPASS WITH HEPARIN COATED EQUIPMENT

Heparin coated heat-exchanger/oxygenator structures were studied in parallel to the above-mentioned experiments. Initially, Duraflo II heparin coated hollow fiber membrane oxygenators were studied without systemic heparinization in an open chest canine model and compared to standard membrane and bubble oxygenators with full systemic heparinization.[12] Besides the fact that the heparin coated oxygenators functioned well over the 6 hour test period, reduced blood loss was the most striking finding for this group perfused without systemic heparinization. Intact hemostasis was also the reason for reduced plasma hemoglobin production for the group perfused without systemic heparinization as cardiotomy suction for mediastinal shed blood recovery was not necessary in this group. Prolonged extracorporeal membrane oxygenation as performed by Toomasian[13] and ourselves, as well as comparison with other commercially available oxygenation devices[14] in varying animal models with different heparinization regimens[15] confirmed the significant improvements in thromboresistance achievable through heparin surface coating of oxygenators and other perfusion devices.

CLINICAL APPLICATION OF HEPARIN COATED LEFT HEART BYPASS EQUIPMENT

With the increasing confidence obtained in our experimental work using heparin coated perfusion equipment and reduced systemic heparinization, clinical application was started. As outlined above, roller-pump left heart bypass for proximal unloading and distal protection during repair of descending thoracic and thoraco-abdominal aortic aneurysms was initiated to improve shunt flow while the aorta is cross-clamped.[16] At that time, a bolus of 5000 IU of heparin (Liquemin, Roche, Basel, Switzerland) was given prior cannulation. If clots were observed in the surgical field, an additional heparin bolus was given. In order to simplify the perfusion procedure, heparin surface coated centrifugal pump heads were introduced after experimental evaluation allowing for non-occlusive pumping during the surgical procedures. No thromboembolic events were observed in these early cases perfused with heparin coated equipment and low systemic heparinization.

CLINICAL APPLICATION OF HEPARIN COATED PARTIAL CARDIOPULMONARY BYPASS

The extremely poor pulmonary function of some patients undergoing repair of the thoracoabdominal aorta with predictable severe problems during single lung ventilation prompted us to add a heparin coated oxygenator to the perfusion circuit. Despite the low systemic heparinization used, these oxygenators remained fully functional throughout the procedures and were macroscopically clean thereafter. Hence, this experience confirmed the results reported for heparin coated equipment used for extracorporeal lung assist.[17]

Partial cardiopulmonary bypass using heparin coated equipment with low systemic heparinization has since been used routinely for proximal unloading and distal support during repair of descending thoracic and thoracoabdominal aortic aneurysms at our institution.[18,19] The overall experience of patients perfused with low systemic heparinization during resection of descending thoracic and thoraco-abdominal aortic aneurysms as well as the details of the procedures are published elsewhere.[20]

Table 1. Selected Heparin and Protamine Doses

	ACT>180 sec	ACT>480 sec
Heparin priming dose	1000 IU/L	5000 IU/L
Heparin loading dose	100 IU/kg b.w.	300 IU/kg b.w.
Criterion for adding heparin	ACT<180s	ACT<480s
Additional heparin dose	2000 IU	5000 IU
Protamine equivalent	100 IU/kg b.w.	300 IU/kg b.w.
Additional protamine titrated according to	ACT	ACT

ACT = activated coagulation time (measured with Hemochron; International Technidyne Inc., Edison, NJ, USA)

CLINICAL APPLICATION OF HEPARIN COATED EQUIPMENT FOR TOTAL CARDIOPULMONARY BYPASS

Further steps in clinical perfusion with heparin coated equipment, at our institution, include total CPB with low systemic heparin for myocardial revascularization. Twenty-two patients undergoing elective coronary artery revascularization were randomly assigned to two groups perfused with heparin coated cardiopulmonary bypass equipment and either low systemic heparinization (ACT greater than 180 sec) or full systemic heparinization (ACT greater than 480 sec) as shown in Table 1.

Inclusion criteria for this study[18] were body weight greater than 50 kg, left ventricular ejection fraction greater than 35 percent, and expected hematocrit value during cardiopulmonary bypass greater than 20%. All patients were successfully revascularized and all perfusion devices functioned well. There was no difference between groups with regard to the pressure gradients measured between inlet and outlet of the oxygenators. However, there was a significant reduction of heparin given to the group perfused with low systemic heparinization which required only 15 percent of the control group. Likewise, the protamine dose for the low heparin group

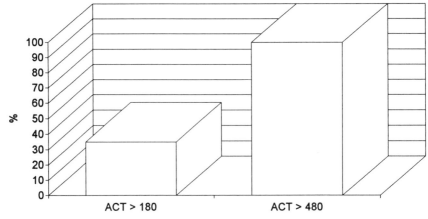

Figure 8. Postoperative blood loss for selected patients perfused with low systemic heparinization as compared to full systemic heparinization.

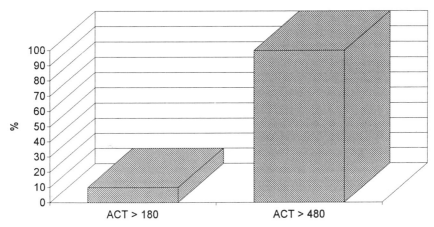

Figure 9. Postoperative transfusion requirements for selected patients perfused with low systemic heparinization as compared to full systemic heparinization.

was 25 percent of control. In the group perfused with low systemic heparinization, blood loss was 35 percent of control (Figure 8) and transfusion requirements accounted for 10 percent of control (Figure 9). Similar results were reported by others.[21]

Heparin coated perfusion equipment was also used under exceptional circumstances for clinical cardiopulmonary bypass without systemic heparinization. The indication for this application was rewarming in accidental deep hypothermia, cardiopulmonary arrest and craniocerebral trauma or polytrauma. Although, we have one long-term survivor without neurological sequelae in this group, this patient group remains difficult.

OVERALL CLINICAL EXPERIENCE WITH HEPARIN COATED EQUIPMENT

Our overall experience with heparin coated equipment used for clinical perfusion is summarized in Table 2. A large part of our knowledge was achieved in proximal unloading and distal perfusion during repair of descending thoracic aortic aneurysms. Following a relatively modest series of 13 patients assisted with left heart bypass, partial cardiopulmonary bypass was used in 38 patients. With the advent of relatively thromboresistant heparin coated cardiotomy reservoirs[22] these devices were added to the pump oxygenator and cardiotomy suction was used clinically with low systemic heparinization[23] in 26 patients. The apparent increase of mortality for patients operated upon with cardiotomy suction (11 percent) as compared to patients operated with an autotransfusion device and no cardiotomy (5 percent) is due to the increased complexity of the lesions operated. As outlined in Table 2, the proportion of ruptured descending thoracic aortic aneurysms was 8 percent in the left heart bypass group, 9 percent in the partial cardiopulmonary bypass group without cardiotomy suction and 35 percent in the partial cardiopulmonary bypass group with cardiotomy suction ($p<0.01$).

Table 2. Total Experience

	Heparin IU	ACT sec	Patient n	Patient x/n	Mortality %
Surgery of descending thoracic aorta					
LHBP with low systemic heparinization (ruptured aneurysms 1/13:8%)	5000	180	13	2/13	15
Partial CPB with low systemic hepatization (ruptured aneurysms 3/38:8%*)	100/kg	180	38	2/38	5
Partial CPB, low systemic heparin and cardiotomy (ruptured aneurysms 9/26:35%*)	100/kg	180	26	3/26	11
Rewarming in accidental deep hypothermia with polytrauma					
Total CPB without systemic heparin	0	120	3	2/3	66
Open heart surgery					
Total CPB with full systemic heparin	300/kg	480	38	0/38	0
Total CPB with low systemic heparin	100/kg	180	43	0/43	0
Total CPB with full systemic heparin and cardiotomy	300/kg	480	9	0/8	0
Total CPB, low systemic heparin and cardiotomy	100/kg	180	12	0/13	0
Overall			182	9/163	5

*$p<0.01$ for comparison between groups (Fisher's test for 2 by 2 tables)

Accidental deep hypothermia combined with trauma remains a difficult clinical problem. Although the 3 patients were rewarmed without technical problems and their hearts resumed spontaneous activity, we have only one long-term survivor.

The group undergoing open heart surgery with heparin coated equipment includes patients undergoing heart surgery within a randomized trial and either full or low systemic heparinization as well as patients perfused with low systemic heparinization refusing transfusion of homologous blood and blood products for various reasons such as Jehovah's witness. The fact that most patients operated on were selected in compliance with a study protocol may explain the very low mortality rate in the subgroups perfused with full systemic heparinization (0/47;0%) as compared to the subgroups perfused with low systemic heparinization (0/55;0%).

In conclusion, perfusion with less systemic heparin can be realized in selected patients by the means of heparin coated equipment. Improved hemostasis, reduced blood loss and transfusion requirements as well as better hemodynamics are the main benefits of this approach. Other groups reported for perfusion with heparin coated equipment reduced activation of complement and other mediators,[24,25] which may decrease the *whole body inflammatory response* linked to cardiopulmonary bypass with standard equipment.

However, it has to be reminded, that the antithrombotic activity of heparin bonded to blood exposed surfaces is strictly flow dependent and requires adequate levels of antithrombin III in the perfusate. Venting of cannulas into the venous line before onset of bypass, immediate recirculation through a shunt in the surgeons field after weaning from bypass, and full systemic heparinization in case of unforeseen problems that might require temporary standstill of the pump are recommended. Non-responding ACT after proper injection of heparin should be treated with a supplement of antithrombin III or fresh-frozen plasma and not exclusively with additional heparin.

REFERENCES

1. McLean J: The thromboplastic action of cephalin. Amer J Physiol 1916;41:250–257.
2. Gibbon JH: Application of mechanical heart and lung apparatus to cardiac surgery. Minnesota Med 1954;37:171.
3. Gott VL, Whiffen JD, Datton RC: Heparin bonding on colloidal graphite surfaces. Science 1963;142:1297–1298.
4. Gott VL: Heparinized shunts for thoracic aortic aneurysms. Ann Thorac Surg 1972;14:219–220.
5. Balding D, Clarke RC: An analysis on performance characteristics for the AF1040C and AF1040 Duraflo heparin coated arterial filters. 11 Journées du CECEC Paris 20–21.6.1986, Abstractbook:23.
6. von Segesser L: Arterial grafting for myocardial revascularization. Springer, Berlin, New York, 1990:39.
7. Weiss BM, von Segesser L, Vetter W, et al: Heparin coated left heart bypass: Renal function and hormonal response. Int J Artif Org 1991;14:792–799.
8. Larm O, Larsson R, Olsson P: A new non-thrombogenic surface prepared by selective covalent binding of heparin via a modified reducing terminal residue. Biomat Med Dev Art Org 1983;11:161–173.
9. von Segesser LK, Weiss BM, Gallino A, et al: Superior hemodynamics in left heart bypass without systemic heparinization. Eur J Cardio-thorac Surg 1990;4:384–389.
10. von Segesser LK, Schilling J, Leskosek B, et al: Morphometric evaluation of heparin coated surfaces after left heart bypass without systemic heparinization: A scanning electron microscopic study. Fourth World Biomaterials Congress, Berlin, April 24–28, Proceedings:9.
11. von Segesser LK, Lachat M, Gallino A, et al: Performance characteristics of centrifugal pumps with heparin surface coating. Thorac Cardiovasc Surg 1990;38:224–228.
12. von Segesser LK, Turina MI: Heparin coated hollow fiber oxygenator without systemic heparinization in comparison to classic membrane and bubble oxygenators. J Extracorp Technol (Proceedings issue)1988:76–80.
13. Toomasian JM, Li-Chen H, Hirschl RB, et al: Evaluation of Duraflo II heparin coating in prolonged extracorporeal membrane oxygenation. ASAIO Transactions 1988;34:410–414.
14. von Segesser LK, Turina M: Cardiopulmonary bypass without systemic heparinization: Performance of heparin coated oxygenators in comparison to classic membrane and bubble oxygenators. J Thorac Cardiovasc Surg 1989;98:386–396.
15. von Segesser L, Lachat M, Leskosek B, et al: Cardiopulmonary bypass with low systemic heparinization: An experimental study. Perfusion 1990;5:267–276.
16. von Segesser LK, Weiss BM, Turina MI: Perfusion with heparin coated equipment: Potential for clinical use. Semin Thorac Cardiovasc Surg 1990;2:373–380.
17. Bindslev L, Eklund J, Norlander O, et al: Treatment of acute respiratory failure by extracorporeal carbon dioxide elimination performed with a surface heparinized artificial lung. Anesthesiology 1987;67:117–120.
18. von Segesser LK, Weiss BM, Garcia E, von Felton A, Turina MI: Reduction and elimination of systemic heparinization during cardiopulmonary bypass. J Thorac Cardiovasc Surg 1992;103:790–799.
19. von Segesser LK, Burki H, Schneider K, Siebenmann R, Schmid ER, Turina M: Outcome and risk factors in surgery of descending thoracic aneurysms. Eur J Cardio-thorac Surg 1988;2:100–105.

20. von Segesser LK, Killer I, Jenni R, et al: Improved distal circulatory support for repair of descending thoracic aortic aneurysms. Ann Thorac Surg 1993;56:1373–80.
21. Aranki SF, Adams DH, Rizzo RJ, et al: Femoral veno-arterial extracorporeal life support with minimal or no heparin. Ann Thorac Surg 1993;56:149–155.
22. von Segesser LK, Pasic M, Leskosek B, Garcia E, Turina M: Heparin coated cardiotomy reservoirs with improved thromboresistance. Cah CECEC 1991;36:9–16.
23. von Segesser LK, Weiss BM, Garcia E, Turina MI: Cardiotomy suction versus red cell spinning during thoracic aortic aneurysms. J Extracorp Technol 1993;25:47–52.
24. Videm V, Svennevig JL, Fosse E, et al: Reduced complement activation with heparin coated oxygenator and tubings in coronary bypass operations. J Thorac Cardiovasc Surg 1992;103:806–813.
25. Gu YJ, van Oeveren W, Akkerman C, et al: Heparin coated circuits reduce the inflammatory response to cardiopulmonary bypass. Ann Thorac Surg 1993;55:917–922.

BLOOD CONSERVATION IN CARDIAC SURGERY

John W. Hammon, Jr., M.D.

Bowman Gray School of Medicine
Winston-Salem, North Carolina

Heightened public concern regarding the incidence of infectious disease related to blood transfusion associated with surgical operations, has recently led to intensified scrutiny of intraoperative transfusion decisions. Surgeons and anesthesiologists, long accustomed to independent decision making, increasingly find their transfusion practices second guessed by blood bank physicians and hospital transfusion committees. To complicate the issue, patients undergoing cardiac surgery in the present era tend to be older, sicker, and with more concurrent conditions requiring well considered decisions regarding transfusion.

The increasing use of multiple blood components and the avoidance of homologous transfusion with whole blood has had the effect of increasing patient exposure to infectious disease. Whole blood transfusion, once common, is approaching obsolescence in many areas with blood component therapy being driven by clinical protocols that, in many cases, have not been proven to be of value. It is the purpose of this chapter to illustrate current practice as well as the risks, benefits, and cost of transfusion. Practical approaches to reduced transfusion requirements such as conduct in the operating room, pharmacologic management, and the role of blood substitutes will be outlined.

TRANSFUSION

The oxygen carrying effects of whole blood, its buffering capacity and properties of volume expansion are well known. However, each transfusion carries with it the risk of complications including febrile reaction (1:100), hemolytic, nonfatal reaction (1:25,000), and hemolytic fatal reaction (<1:1,000,000). More serious are the delayed infectious reaction such as HIV-1 (1:40,000–150,000), $HTLV_1$ (<1:100,000), hepatitis B (<1:250.000), hepatitis C (1:500–3,000), and cytomegalovirus (approximately 0.9 percent in immuno-competent recipient).

The average number of units of blood transfusion post cardiac surgery was 9 units between 1969–1971, 4.7 units/patient in 1977, and 2.9 units in 1991.[1] The transfusion requirement is significantly increased in patients requiring re-operation following coronary bypass (4.1±5.1 units/patient). Preoperative red cell volume and the need for re-operation have been identified as the best predictors for the need of transfusion in cardiac surgery.[2] One recent study indicated that 143 (6.1 percent) required re-operation for bleeding in a review of 2,355 open heart surgery patients.[3] The incidence of bleeding in open heart surgery contrasts with the much lower incidence of hemorrhagic complications in general surgery, reported to be a little over 2 percent.[4]

The emphasis on safety of blood transfusions has created an environment in which costs have become increasingly important. Forbes et al.[5] estimated that the cost to transfuse a unit of blood was $155.00 in 1989. The acquisition cost was $57.00 (37 percent). The handling, laboratory and administration cost was $98.00 (63 percent). In recent years, the average red cell price has increased from $48.00 in 1988 to $65.00 per unit in 1992, a 35 percent increase. Based on this inflationary trend, the transfusion cost would be approximately $210.00 in 1993. With the increased risk associated with blood transfusions and the economic implications, a blood conservation program in cardiac surgery becomes a practical necessity.

Operating Room Practices

Any blood conservation program will fail unless the operating team pays attention to a number of small but important details. It is very important that the surgical team technically control most bleeding so that blood is not exposed to cardiotomy suction. The use of this blood retrieval system activates platelets, causes hemolysis and white cell destruction and increases post pump bleeding. The use of low-flow cardiopulmonary bypass or circulatory arrest techniques limits exposure of blood elements to bypass circuits and thus can decrease bleeding. Although cooling the patient can inactivate platelets, hypothermia allows lower bypass flows and thus damages blood elements less.

Reducing the transfusion trigger to a hemoglobin level of 6 g/dL on bypass and 8 g/dL thereafter, has been shown to reduce transfusion requirements without jeopardizing surgical success.[6] This formula may have to be modified in older, more high-risk patients.

Autologous Pre-Donation

The rationale for this procedure is that the patient donate his own blood repeatedly while awaiting elective surgery. Although this method has very sound and attractive features, the current practice of cardiac surgery in this country clearly is being directed toward a rapid response system in which a delay of 3 weeks for most patients requiring cardiac surgery would be unacceptable to physicians and patients alike. If the avoidance of allogeneic transfusion is the goal, it has been shown that obtaining three or more units from patients was critical.[7] This provided a three week donation schedule to obtain three units of autologous blood. In 1992, 50 percent of the coronary bypass patients at Bowman Gray School of Medicine underwent cardiac catheterization and surgery on the same admission with a mean interval of 4.1 days between these two interventions. Surprisingly, this proportion was almost identical for coronary artery bypass grafting patients and for patients undergoing cardiac valve replacement or repair. Over half of the patients discharged between cardiac catheterization and surgery were then readmitted for surgery within two weeks. If three weeks represents the optimal preoperative period for autologous blood donation, then approximately 10 percent of our cardiac surgery patients would have had sufficient time to donate three units while meeting usual eligibility requirements for pre-donation.

In addition, there are some risks to waiting for elective coronary revascularization. A mortality of 2.2 percent occurred on a 90 day waiting list in European report.[8] Brittain and colleagues[9] reported that 11.5 percent of their pre-donation patients had to discontinue donations, predominantly because of increasing angina. It seems to be clear that autologous pre-donation is not feasible in the current climate for cardiac surgery in this country; however, if cost containment procedures mandate a more elective surgery profile in the future, autologous pre-donation will have to be reconsidered.

Intraoperative Pre-bypass Blood Conservation

Intraoperative withdrawal of whole blood or platelet-rich plasma before cardiopulmonary bypass has also been recommended as a strategy to reduce exposure to allogeneic transfusions and possibly to decrease blood loss after cardiopulmonary bypass. Pre-bypass whole blood withdrawal offers significant theoretical benefits. Because cardiopulmonary bypass either damages or consumes platelets and causes some hemolysis, preservation of platelets and red cells by withdrawing and storing whole blood makes sense. Unfortunately, studies have not proved definitively that withdrawing a unit or more of whole blood and then hemodiluting the patient to maintain blood volume reduces postoperative transfusion requirements.[10] In addition, other authors have found that withdrawal of whole blood prior to bypass can cause problems in some patients. Patients with impaired left ventricular function have had evidence of adverse hemodynamic consequences of whole blood withdrawal prior to bypass and other patients with unstable angina have shown evidence of ST segment depression during hemodilution.[11]

Our own experience at this institution suggests that the use of pre-cardiopulmonary bypass whole blood withdrawal predisposes to excessive hemodilution. This requires that the surgical team accept very low hemoglobin levels or raise the transfusion trigger.

The withdrawal of autologous platelet-rich plasma by plasmapheresis during induction of anesthesia and while preparing the patient for bypass is another attractive theoretical maneuver. Unfortunately, only one study using tightly controlled scientific method and transfusion trigger supports the use of platelet rich plasma in reducing allogeneic transfusion.[12] The equipment is expensive and requires trained personnel for its use. In 1987, a consensus conference on platelet transfusion therapy concluded that "There is no justification for prophylactic platelet administration in patients undergoing cardiac surgery."[13] Using their findings and common sense, it would appear that most patients undergoing cardiac surgery do not require platelet or autologous whole blood administration in order to reduce transfusion requirements.

Operative and Postoperative Blood Salvage

Salvage and processing techniques of the blood remaining in the extracorporeal circuit after cardiopulmonary bypass continue to be a subject of great interest. In the early 70's, blood remaining in the extracorporeal circuit was administered directly to the patient after cardiopulmonary bypass. This direct infusion of a large volume of diluted blood required that the patient have adequate cardiac and renal function to accommodate the increased volume load. Addressing this problem, centrifugation techniques were developed in which the diluted blood remaining in the extracorporeal circuit was centrifuged and washed, resulting in a red blood suspension relatively free of heparin, plasma free hemoglobin and other solutes. Although the red cells are retained, the less dense components of blood, such as plasma proteins, platelets and coagulation factors, are discarded.

Another means by which cardiopulmonary circuit blood can be processed is by ultrafiltration. Ultrafiltration uses trans-membrane pressure to remove plasma water from the cellular elements in plasma proteins. The advantage of ultrafiltration is that both the plasma proteins and the red blood cells are salvaged. Disadvantages of this method can include exposure of the blood to high trans-membrane pressures which can cause hemolysis and heparin concentration, requiring extra amounts of protamine for reversal. In addition, withdrawing excessive amounts of water from the bypass circuit concentrates the volume in the circuit, making withdrawal from bypass, in some cases, difficult.

Numerous studies have been performed to try to ascertain which one of the previous three methods has the advantage in reducing allogeneic transfusion following cardiopulmonary bypass. Suffice it to say that all three techniques are advantageous and reduce allogeneic transfusion and no one of the three offers a clear advantage.[14]

PHARMACOLOGIC AGENTS AND BLOOD SUBSTITUTES

Certain pharmacologic products, notably desmopressin (DDAVP) antifibrinolytic medications, and protease inhibitors (aprotinin), now constitute adjunctive therapy for the control of bleeding during and after cardiac surgery. Recombinant human erythropoietin (RHE) has been used to increase the synthesis of red cells prior to surgery and certain colloids and blood substitutes have been used as adjuncts to transfusion. We will discuss these agents in regards to blood conservation related to cardiac surgery.

Desmopressin

Normal functioning of the coagulation cascade depends on adequate plasma concentration of Factor VIII. Persistence of Factor VIII in plasma requires von Willebrand's factor (vWF). DDAVP, an analog of vasopressin, lacking in vasoconstrictor activity alters coagulation by its effect on circulatory endothelial cells and platelets. Infusion of desmopressin in pharmacologic doses causes vWF to be released from storage sites into plasma. This has a procoagulant effect and increases platelet aggregation. There are no important side effects from the administration of DDAVP, although plasma levels of tissue plasminogen activator (t-PA) increase after the administration of desmopressin which has the theoretical effect of worsening bleeding in some patients.[15]

Desmopressin is the drug of choice for bleeding crises in patients with uremia and cirrhosis. In addition, desmopressin can correct the bleeding time abnormality in patients taking aspirin.[16] Interest in prophylactic desmopressin's hemostatic potential in cardiac surgery stems from the known acquired platelet abnormalities and theoretical salutary effects of increased vWF on platelet adhesion and in shortening prolonged bleeding time. Salzman and colleagues[17] initially reported a marked reduction in bleeding after bypass in patients undergoing cardiac procedures known for excessive postoperative bleeding. Subsequent investigations have not reproduced these results and the exact role of desmopressin in cardiac surgical patients is, at the moment, conjectural.[18] The role of desmopressin in cardiac surgery patients receiving preoperative platelet antagonists has not been carefully studied and therefore its potential in these groups awaits analysis.

Synthetic Antifibrinolytics

Fibrinolysis may commonly accompany cardiac surgery using cardiopulmonary bypass. When excessive fibrinolysis overwhelms the ability of plasma binding substances and fibrin split products are released into the circulation, these interfere with future clot formation and can increase surgical bleeding. Inhibitors of fibrinolysis, which are analogs of lysine, bind to the kringles of plasminogen or plasmin at their lysine binding sites, displacing plasminogen from the fibrin molecular surface and thus interfering with plasmin's ability to split fibrinogen. Epsilon-amino caproic acid (EACA) and tranexamic acid are both examples of these compounds.

Tranexamic acid is approximately ten times as potent as EACA. The side effects of antifibrinolytics may be related to absolute dose administered.[19] Thus, the therapeutic index of tranexamic acid is more favorable than that of EACA. Patients with bleeding in the kidneys or ureters may thrombose the upper urinary tract due to the urinary concentration of antifibrinolytic drug. Although the theoretically greater risk of a systemic thrombosis is superficially supported by anecdotal reports of intracranial and other vascular thromboses, controlled studies do not support this contention.[20] Disseminated intravascular coagulation constitutes a contraindication to antifibrinolytic therapy, lest the intravascular clot so formed, remain intact.

Fibrinolysis may commonly accompany extracorporeal circulation.[21] Contact activation of Factor XII may account for part of this lytic state by directly activating plasminogen and by inducing thrombin formation via the coagulation cascade. EACA has been used for years to try to decrease excessive postoperative bleeding after cardiac surgery with conflicting results.[22] In more recent studies, EACA has been given in prophylactic doses to theoretically bind platelet receptors responsible for platelet activation during cardiopulmonary bypass. This then reduced the number of activated platelets with a salutary effect on postoperative bleeding.[23] Several studies have now appeared in the literature supporting the use of prophylactic EACA and more recently, tranexamic acid and with generally positive results in reducing postoperative bleeding.[24]

Aprotinin

Aprotinin (Trasylol®, Miles Inc., West Haven, CT), currently isolated from bovine lung, is a serine protease inhibitor which has been in clinical use outside the United States for more than 35 years for a variety of indications, including pancreatitis, shock, and fibrinolysis. Recently, however, this polypeptide has generated great interest for its apparent ability to decrease blood loss during cardiac surgery. The specific mechanisms responsible for this potential beneficial effect include the inhibition of plasmin and kallikrein[25] and platelet preservation by binding to platelet membrane receptors.[26]

Because aprotinin is a polypeptide, anaphylactic reactions have been reported.[27] Allergic reactions are much more likely in patients previously exposed to the drug. However, the overall incidence of aprotinin allergy appears to be less than 0.1 percent. The potential for renal toxicity because of aprotinin strong affinity for renal tissue, is not surprising. Despite animal experiments showing renal toxicity in high doses, the effect on humans has shown surprisingly few renal events.[28] The use of Aprotinin in cardiac surgery is not new. However, the most dramatic results have been from several recent well controlled, prospective studies demonstrating large decreases in post-cardiopulmonary bypass blood loss and significant reduction in blood bank products used in patients receiving aprotinin.[25,29,30] Compared with earlier studies, these reports have used larger doses of aprotinin. Drug administration has consisted of an intravenous bolus following anesthesia induction, continuous intravenous infusion for the duration of the operation, and a bolus added to the pump prime. Only one study shows a potential for thrombosis in coronary bypass grafts.[31] The remainder of the studies demonstrate no increase in myocardial infarction postoperatively.

Of special interest is heparin management during cardiopulmonary bypass in patients receiving aprotinin. This drug inhibits activation of both the extrinsic clotting cascade and platelets and increases the activated clotting time (ACT).[30] Prolongation of the ACT with aprotinin has been mistakenly attributed to improvement in anticoagulation during bypass with a possible benefit in reduction of heparin dose.[32] Unfortunately, this prolongation is artifactual and other methods of monitoring anticoagulation during bypass are necessary. Under no circumstances can heparin dose be reduced, and reversion to an empirical dosing regimen is necessary, maintaining an ACT of greater than 750 seconds with mild hypothermia. Newer measures of heparin activity and thrombin inhibition are being developed which will make the administration of aprotinin safer in the presence of heparin and extracorporeal circulation.

Cost

Any prophylactic therapy to reduce cardiopulmonary bypass associated bleeding entails costs to prevent presumed complications. Factors that will determine the appropriateness of pharmaceuticals to prevent bleeding include the cost of the drug, the expected savings in terms of blood loss and transfusion prevented, and the estimated adverse outcome from omission of prophylaxis. In the case of aprotinin, Canadian data predict that a prophylactic course will cost over 100 times that of EACA.[33] Routine aprotinin administration to all patients undergoing coronary bypass surgery in the United States could increase yearly costs by about $300,000,000 (300,000 procedures at $1,000 each). Indeed, even routine EACA prophylaxis could increase the health care bill for coronary bypass by $1,000,000. Very careful cost/benefit ratios will have to be calculated for all of these procedures before routine prophylaxis can be advised. In the meantime, there is no doubt that antifibrinolytics offer significant advantage in some groups of patients to correct cardiopulmonary bypass-induced coagulopathy and have an important role in the armamentarium in the cardiac health care team.

Recombinant Human Erythropoietin

Erythropoietin, a glycoprotein hormone normally produced by the kidney in response to tissue hypoxia, stimulates bone marrow erythroid colony-forming units to divide and produce proerythroblasts, which give rise to mature red blood cells. The gene for erythropoietin has been cloned and the hormone can now be produced in pharmacologic quantities with recombinant DNA techniques. Human volunteers respond vigorously to RHE with an increase in hemoglobin, hematocrit and reticulocyte count, provided there is adequate serum iron to support increased erythropoiesis.[34] The drug can be administered by a variety of routes, but intravenous administration provides the most active red cell synthesis. An occasional patient with impaired renal function can experience central nervous system complications with RHE administration. Normal volunteers have only experienced mild complications.

The minimum period of time to substantially decrease postoperative transfusion requirements in surgical patients is approximately 14 days. Intravenous administration of the drug can reduce this time to approximately 7 days in some patients. For this reason, the drug has the same theoretical disadvantages as autologous transfusion in that the vast majority of cardiac surgical patient are now operated on an urgent or semi-elective basis precluding a two week wait for optimum effect of the drug. Studies with combined erythropoietin and autologous donation have not been performed but offer a theoretical benefit in reducing the time for donation of autologous blood and preventing many of the anemia related complications during autologous pre-donation.[35]

Blood Substitutes

The ideal blood substitute should be able to support oxygen and carbon dioxide, providing buffering and free radical quenching, expand intravascular volume and maintain colloid osmotic pressure. It should also be non-toxic, non-pyrogenic, sterile and non-allergenic and have reasonable persistence in the intravascular space.

Perfluorocarbons

Fluosol-DA 20 percent (Alpha Therapeutic Inc., Los Angeles, CA) was proposed and tested in humans and found to be relatively non-toxic, although some anaphylactic reactions were observed. However, a typical dose of this synthetic fluorocarbon (20 mL/kg) requires a high arterial oxygen tension to carry less than 3 vol% of oxygen; thus, oxygen delivery is inadequate for Fluosol-DA to serve as a total hemoglobin substitute.[36] A new fluorocarbon, perfluorooctyl bromide (Oxygent™, Alliance Pharmaceutical Corp., San Diego, CA) which can be administered in a 50 percent solution has a clinical efficacy much improved over that of Fluosol-DA.[37] Persistence in the blood stream continues for 24 to 48 hours with Oxygent™, thus limiting its usefulness as a complete blood substitute. However, this same limitation can also be expected for all currently experimental blood substitutes.

Hemoglobin Solutions

Hemoglobin solutions have the potential to meet most specifications for the ideal blood substitute. For the last twenty years, many approaches to obtaining pure hemoglobin have been tried and recent developments are encouraging. In the last several years, small doses of purified hemoglobin solutions have been infused into humans with good results, although not in clinically relevant doses.[38] Pertinent issues about hemoglobin solutions that must still be addressed are: oxygen affinity and cooperatively, intravascular half-life, auto-oxidation, colloid osmotic pressure, polymerization techniques, cost/benefit ratios and clinical indications.

For the short term, blood substitutes will remain in the research area. Bovine derived polymerized hemoglobin may emerge as the most practical product if it maintains its low renal toxicity and benign immunologic profile in continued human testing.

SUMMARY

In conclusion, the various modalities available to the cardiac surgical team to reduce allogeneic transfusion have been reviewed. What, then, comprises an effective regimen for cardiac surgical blood conservation in the 1990's? Many possibilities exist but three strategies best balance efficacy, practicality, risk and cost: 1) intra-operative red blood cell salvage, including the residual contents of the extracorporeal circuit, 2) acceptance of low hemoglobin levels (6.0 g/dL during CPB and 8.0 g/dL postoperatively) when the patient possesses the hemodynamic capacity to compensate adequately for this level of anemia, even if modest inotropic assistance is required, and 3) prophylactic administration of antifibrinolytic drugs (EACA) during cardiopulmonary bypass to patients at high risk for post-cardiopulmonary bypass hemorrhage, and possibly even for all cardiac surgical patients.

REFERENCES

1. Increasing the safety of blood transfusions, The American Red Cross, Washington, DC 1992.
2. Bayer WL, Coenen WM, Jenkins DC, Zucker ML: The use of blood and blood components in 1769 patients undergoing open heart surgery. Ann Thorac Surg 1980;29:117–21.
3. Cosgrove DL, Loop FD, Lytle BW, et al: Determinants of blood utilization during myocardial revascularization. Ann Thorac Surg 1985;40:380–4.
4. Papa MZ, Amsterdam E, Schneiderman J, et al: Hemorrhagic complication encountered on a surgical service. Am J Surg 1984;147:378–81.
5. Forbes JM, Anderson GF, Bleeker FC, et al: Blood transfusion costs: a multicenter study. Transfusion 1992;31:318–23.
6. Robertie PG, Gravlee GP: Safe limits of isovolemic hemodilution and recommendations for erythrocyte transfusion. Int Anesthesiol Clin 1990;28:197–204.
7. Owings DV, Kruskall MS, Thurer RL, Donovan LM: Autologous blood donations prior to elective cardiac surgery - safety and effect on subsequent blood use. JAMA 1989;262:1963–68.
8. Suttorp MJ, Kingma JH, Vos J, et al: Determinants for early mortality in patients awaiting coronary artery bypass graft surgery: a case-control study. Eur Heart J 1992;13:238–42.
9. Britton LW, Eastlund T, Dziuban SW, et al: Predonated autologous blood use in elective cardiac surgery. Ann Thorac Surg 1989;47:529–32.
10. Gravlee, GP: Autologous blood collection is useful for elective coronary artery bypass graft surgery. Cardiothorac Vasc Anesth 1994;8:238–241.
11. Kruskall MS, Glazer EE, Leonard SS, et al: Utilization and effectiveness of a hospital autologous preoperative blood donor program. Transfusion 1986;26:335–40.
12. DelRossi AJ, Cernaianu AC, Vertrees RA, et al: Platelet-rich plasma reduces postoperative blood loss after cardiopulmonary bypass. J Thorac Cardiovasc Surg 1990;100:281–6.
13. Consensus Conference: Platelet transfusion therapy. JAMA 1987;257:1777–80.
14. Sutton RG, Kratz JM, Spinale FG, Crawford FA: Comparison of three blood-processing techniques during and after cardiopulmonary bypass. Ann Thorac Surg 1993;56:938–43.
15. Colman RW, Hirsh J, Marder VJ, Salzman EW, eds: Hemostasis and thrombosis. 2nd ed. Philadelphia: Lippincott, 1987:86–88, 1033–1034.
16. Mannucci PM, Vicente V, Vianello L, et al: Controlled trial of desmopressin in liver cirrhosis and other conditions associated with a prolonged bleeding time. Blood 1986;67:1148–53.
17. Salzman EW, Weinstein MJ, Weintraub RM, et al: Treatment with desmopressin acetate to reduce blood loss after cardiac surgery. N Engl J Med 1986;314:1402–1406.
18. Hackmann T, Gascoyne RD, Naiman SC, et al: A trial of desmopressin (l-desamino-8-D-arginine vasopressin) to reduce blood loss in uncomplicated cardiac surgery. N Engl J Med 1989;321:1437–43.
19. Verstraete M: Clinical application of inhibitors of fibrinolysis. Drugs 1985;29:236–61.
20. Vinnicombe J, Shuttleworth KED: Aminocaproic acid in the control of haemorrhage after prostatectomy. Lancet 1966;1:232–34.
21. Kucuk O, Kwaan HC, Frederickson J, et al: Increased fibrinolysis in patients undergoing cardiopulmonary bypass operation. Am J Hematol 1986;23:223–39.
22. McClure PD, Izsak J: The use of e-aminocaproic acid to reduce bleeding during cardiac bypass in children with congenital heart disease. Anesthesiology 1974;40:604–8.
23. Vander Salm TJ, Ansell JE, Okike ON, et al: The role of E-aminocaproic acid in reducing bleeding after cardiac operation: a double-blind randomized study. J Thorac Cardiovasc Surg 1989;95:538–40.

24. Horrow JC, Hlavacek J, Strong MD, et al: Prophylactic tranexamic acid decreases bleeding after cardiac operations. J Thorac Cardiovasc Surg 1990;99:70–4.
25. Bidstrup BP, Royston D, Sapsford RN, Taylor KM: Reduction in blood loss after cardiopulmonary bypass using high dose aprotinin (trasylol): studies in patients undergoing aortocoronary bypass surgery, reoperations and valve replacement for endocarditis. J Thorac Cardiovasc Surg 1989;97:364–72.
26. Van Oeveren W, Jansen NJ, Bidstrup BP, et al: Effects of aprotinin on hemostatic mechanism during cardiopulmonary bypass. Ann Thorac Surg 1987;44:640–5.
27. Freeman JG, Turner GA, Venables CW, Latner AL: Serial use of aprotinin and incidence of allergic reactions. Curr Med Res Opin 1983;8:559–61.
28. Madeddu P, Oppes M, Soro A, et al: The effects of aprotinin, a kallikrein inhibitor, on renin release and urinary sodium excretion in mild essential hypertension. J Hypertens 1987;5:581–6.
29. Royston D, Bidstrup BP, Taylor KM, Sapsford RN: Effect of aprotinin on need for blood transfusion after repeat open heart surgery. Lancet 1987;2:1289–91.
30. Dietrich W, Barankay A, Dilthey G, et al: Reduction of homologous blood requirement in cardiac surgery by intraoperative aprotinin application: clinical experience in 152 cardiac surgical patient. Thorac Cardiovasc Surg 1989;37:92–8.
31. Cosgrove DM, Heric B, Lytle BW, et al: Aprotinin therapy for reoperative myocardial revascularization: a randomized, double-blind, placebo controlled study. Ann Thorac Surg 1992;54:1031–8.
32. Hunt BJ, Segal H, Yacoub M: Aprotinin and heparin monitoring during cardiopulmonary bypass. Circulation 1992;86 Suppl:II410–II412.
33. Hardy G-F, Deroches J: The usefulness of natural and synthetic antifibrinolytics in cardiac surgery. Can J Anaesth 1992; 353–365.
34. Essers U, Muller W, Pollycove M, et al: Effect of erythropoietin in normal men and in patients with renal insufficiency. Proc Eur Dial Transplant Assoc Eur Ren Assoc 1975;11:389–402.
35. Goodnough LT, Rudnik S, Price TH, Ballas SK, et al: Increased preoperative collection of autologous blood with recombinant human erythropoietin therapy. N Engl J Med 1989;321:1163–8.
36. Gould SA, Rosen AL, Sehgal LR, et al: Fluosol-DA as a red-cell substitute in acute anemia. N Engl J Med 1986;314:1653–56.
37. Long DM, Mattrey RF, Long DC, et al: Overview of experimental and clinical applications of PFOB. Biomater Artif Cells Artif Organs 1987;15:333.
38. Winslow RM: Blood substitutes: current status. Transfusion 1989;29:753–54.

PATIENT SELECTION CRITERIA FOR LEFT VENTRICULAR ASSIST DEVICE PLACEMENT

Mehmet C. Oz, M.D., Howard R. Levin, M.D.,
Keith Reemtsma, M.D., and Eric A. Rose, M.D.

College of Physicians and Surgeons
Columbia University
New York, New York

The incidence of end-stage congestive heart failure is currently estimated at 50,000 cases per year in the United States.[1,2] The majority of these patients are potential heart transplant recipients. The availability of donor organs, however, remains relatively fixed at approximately 2,000 annually.[3] This vast discrepancy has led to the successful development of left ventricular assist devices (LVADs) as a bridge-to-transplantation and has raised the issue of permanent device implantation in lieu of transplantation.[4] Although alternative technologies such as skeletal muscle cardiomyoplasty, cross-species transplantation, and transgenic animal breeding have been proposed, LVADs are the only clinically viable alternative in the near future. In addition to avoiding the immunosuppression complications of transplantation and the long-term limitations posed by accelerated atherosclerosis, LVADs could be produced in the large numbers required by the heart failure population. The limitations of LVADs include their cost, estimated at $50,000 per unit, and their risk of infection, thromboembolism, and mechanical failure.

As in many other novel interventions, success with LVAD placement hinges on correct patient selection. These devices have often been used on patients who are extremely ill, with predictably poor results. The recipient population overlaps with the heart transplant candidate group, and the choice between these two therapies may be difficult. Since organs are a scarce resource, one could view LVADs as first line therapy for patients too ill to undergo heart transplantation, such as patients unable to be weaned from cardiopulmonary bypass. Placement of a short-term device, such as an Abiomed® circuit (Danvers, MA), to allow control of bleeding and evaluation of end-organ dysfunction can be followed by implantation of a long-term implantable device such as the ThermoCardiosystems® unit (Woburn, MA). A second important group would include patients too ill to wait the 6 to 12 months required for heart transplantation. This would include large sized patients with O blood type and patients with a positive reactive antibody titer for whom prospective cross-matching will be required. In addition, some patients will acutely decompensate and be unable to wait for an organ to become available. A third, heretofore avoided group would be patients over the age of 65 who are generally not considered for heart transplantation.

With these three groups in mind, an outline of contraindications to LVAD placement can be generated to avoid the pitfall of device insertion into extraordinarily high risk patients.

Candidates for receipt of a TCI Heartmate® device should be:
1. an approved transplant candidate
2. on inotropic and/or intra-aortic balloon pump support and
3. pulmonary capillary wedge pressure greater than 20 mm Hg with
4. systolic blood pressure less than 80 mm Hg or
5. cardiac index less than 2 L/min/m^2.

We have also implanted LVADs in patients who could not be weaned from cardiopulmonary bypass and are stabilized with use of short-term extracorporeal mechanical circuits such as the Abiomed assist device. Particular attention must be directed towards preserving cerebral and renal function in these unstable patients.

Patients who meet hemodynamic criteria for LVAD support should also be screened for concomitant valvular, coronary, or congenital pathology.

VALVE LESIONS

Aortic regurgitation must be addressed during LVAD insertion. Since the LVAD circuit inflow is from the left ventricular apex and the outflow is to the ascending aorta, a circular flow pattern without peripheral perfusion may be established. Mild-to-moderate aortic insufficiency may become severe after institution of LVAD support since the left ventricular diastolic pressure will be reduced to near 0, thus increasing the transvalvular gradient. In addition, placement of the outflow graft close to the aortic valve may cause turbulence, further worsening aortic insufficiency.

Severe aortic stenosis should always be corrected prior to embarking on any permanent cardiac replacement since these patients often have adequate myocardial reserve, even with preoperative ejection fractions of less than 10 percent and severe congestive heart failure. Lesser degrees of aortic stenosis are probably insignificant if LVAD support is instituted since the aortic valve often opens only during the few seconds of pump venting every 8 hours in most of our patients. Placement of an aortic prosthesis, especially a mechanical type, should be avoided as thromboembolic complications have been reported.

Mitral insufficiency is inconsequential in LVAD patients since the left ventricle is completely evacuated and the left ventricular end diastolic pressure is near 0 mm Hg. Mitral stenosis, if severe, should be corrected.

Tricuspid and pulmonary insufficiency should be corrected since right ventricular function should be optimized at the time of LVAD insertion. Since many of these patients have moderate-to-severe tricuspid regurgitation, we have had a low threshold for tricuspid annuloplasty. To date no significant complications have resulted.

CORONARY ARTERY DISEASE

Patients with inoperable coronary artery disease can continue to have angina and ischemic myocardial injury while on LVAD support. These are manifest hemodynamically by right heart failure and decreased LVAD flow. Continued anti-ischemic regimens are sometimes warranted. If the patient has had previous coronary artery bypass, attempts should be made to preserve already present bypass grafts to avoid right heart failure and arrhythmia associated with ventricular ischemia.

ARRHYTHMIA

Atrial fibrillation will hinder right heart function, but is reasonably well tolerated in the LVAD recipients. Attempts to maintain the patient in sinus rhythm during the early post-operative period are made in order to reduce the risk of serious right heart failure. Long-term anticoagulation is indicated in this sub-set of patients, unlike other LVAD recipients.

Ventricular arrhythmias are commonly encountered in cardiomyopathy patients and continue to occur post LVAD insertion. Although previously felt to be a strict contraindication for univentricular support, we have had no serious hemodynamic compromise associated with ventricular fibrillation after the perioperative period. Our patients have complained only of generalized weakness. We noted a moderate decrease in LVAD flow (1.7 ± 0.75 L/min) with a decrease in mean blood pressure of usually less than 20 percent. Central venous pressure generally remained constant during these episodes. All hemodynamic parameters returned to pre-arrhythmia values upon resolution of the arrhythmia. No significant end-organ injury was evident. Early electrical or pharmacologic cardioversion is warranted to avoid thrombus formation and the theoretical risk of right ventricular injury.

ATRIAL OR VENTRICULAR SEPTAL DEFECTS

Atria or ventricular septal defects should be repaired at the time of LVAD insertion to avoid the right to left shunt and subsequent destruction caused by sudden and permanent reduction in left-sided filling pressures. Intraoperatively measured left atrial and left ventricular pressures are 0 if the LVAD inflow is correctly positioned.

RIGHT HEART FAILURE

Right heart failure is the cause of death in 20 percent of LVAD recipients. Its etiology is not well understood and at times appears without apparent reason, as a right ventricle that can pump successfully against the high pulmonary resistance and left atrial pressure seen in cardiomyopathy patients should function only better if the left atrial pressure is reduced to 0. The loss of a septal contribution to ventricular function observed when the septum is retracted by the suction of the LVAD may play a role. Alternatively, the increase in pulmonary vascular resistance observed following cardiopulmonary bypass (next section) may be the predominant factor. Preoperative right ventricular stroke work does appear to be a major prospective determinant of right ventricular failure. In the 92 TCI recipient patients studied, patients suffering postoperative right heart failure had half (6.3 versus 11.7), the preoperative measured right ventricular stroke work as patients avoiding this complication.

PULMONARY FACTORS

Severe obstructive or restrictive pulmonary disease is a contraindication to LVAD placement since these patients will often desaturate during the perioperative period and need above-average pulmonary reserve. Decreased pulmonary diffusion capacity is often observed in congestive heart failure patients and should not be considered a contraindication.

Increased pulmonary vascular resistance is often encountered; however, if the native right ventricle has tolerated these pressures, it should continue to function well postoperatively. Left atrial pressures are reduced to 0 postoperatively, and the pulmonary vascular resistance of patients on chronic LVAD support tends to decrease. Almost all of the 20 percent of LVAD recipients developing right heart failure do so in the immediate perioperative period. The sudden increase in pulmonary vascular resistance causing this problem is likely a combination of effects from cardiopulmonary bypass and blood product transfusions. Especially in patients with continued bleeding requiring large amounts of blood product infusion, worsening pulmonary hypertension with subsequent right heart failure is the norm.

RENAL FACTORS

Patients should not require dialysis and should have a creatinine level of less than 5 g per 24 hours prior to LVAD insertion. In patients with renal insufficiency, return of renal function is usually seen as systemic pressure increases and the need for inotropic agents is reduced. Early institution of continuous veno-veno or arterio-venous hemofiltration is mandatory in the early postoperative period to facilitate fluid management in these patients. Avoidance of the large fluid shifts encountered with hemodialysis reduces further insults to the kidneys and avoids hemodynamic compromise in these already critically ill patients.

HEPATIC FACTORS

Liver insufficiency with resultant inadequate production of clotting factors can lead to coagulopathy, blood product infusions, pulmonary hypertension, right heart failure and worsening hepatic congestion and failure. Preoperative normalization of coagulation profiles, including a prothrombin time less than 15, and restoration of normal transaminases and bilirubin are essential to successful LVAD insertion. Preoperative blood product administration or intra-aortic balloon pump placement are often necessary to achieve these goals.

Postoperatively, early institution of biventricular support, if right heart failure develops, is mandatory to avoid worsening hepatic congestion and coagulopathy.

INFECTIOUS DISEASE

Most of the morbidity following the immediate post-operative period has involved infection. Since most end-stage heart failure patients develop systemic infection at some point during their illness, we screen these patients carefully for pre-existing evidence for infection. Absence of positive blood cultures, especially for fungus, for one week prior to device insertion is imperative. All previous sources of infection including pneumonia, urinary tract infections, and central venous line infections must be completely resolved. Patients receive preoperative staphylococcus specific and broad spectrum antibiotics as well as anti-fungal prophylactics at the time of device insertion and removal.

MISCELLANEOUS

Additional factors which complicate LVAD insertion and survival with LVAD support include significant blood dyscrasias, co-morbid disease which limits life expectancy to less than 5 years and body surface areas of less than 1.5 m^2. The last restriction is a result of the need to implant the pumping chamber beneath the abdominal wall without causing excessive disruptive force on the wound. Several of our smaller patients have complained of pressure pain resulting from device placement, although none have had wound complications.

As the technology improves and our experience with use of these devices for long-term support increases, willingness to use LVADs as an alternative rather than a bridge-to-transplantation will increase. The patient selection criteria cited in this review may help avoid complications following device insertion and allow maximal utilization of this new intervention.

REFERENCES

1. Smith WM: Epidemiology of congestive heart failure. Am J Cardiol 1985;55:3A.
2. Schocken DD, Arrieta MI, Leaverton PE, Ross EA: Prevalence and mortality rate of congestive heart failure in the United States. JACC 1992;20(2):301–6.
3. Kriett JM, Kaye MP: The Registry of the International Society for Heart and Lung Transplantation. J Heart Lung Trans 1991;10(4):491–498.
4. Oz MC, Levin HR, Rose EA: Wearable left ventricular assist device for long term mechanical circulatory assistance. Cardiac Chronicle 1993;7(7):1–7.

SUPPORT OF THE FAILING HEART BY MECHANICAL DEVICES

William C. DeVries, M.D.

DeVries and Associates
Louisville, Kentucky

It has been estimated that more than 27 million people in the United States are affected by cardiovascular disease with more than 4 million of them involving coronary artery disease. Myocardial infarction claims more than 650,000 lives annually. It is estimated that there are approximately 150,000 cases of cardiogenic shock in the Unites States each year.[1] It has been shown that in spite of pharmacological agents, intra-aortic balloon pumping, and emergency coronary revascularization, the overall mortality of cardiogenic shock still remains 70 to 90 percent. The limited use of left ventricular assist devices and mechanical support of the ventricle has significantly decreased the mortality of cardiogenic shock. Many studies have shown that myocardial ischemia, which is a resulting etiology of the severe dysfunction found in cardiogenic shock, may be reversible. Moreover, myocardial dysfunction post cardiopulmonary bypass can be reversed with pharmacological support and mechanical circulatory support.[2] The work of Pae[3] demonstrates that a satisfactory quality of life post discharge and long-term survival may be achieved in these patients who have been in cardiogenic shock and required ventricular mechanical support for survival.

The Institute of Medicine estimates that approximately 35,000 to 75,000 patients may require circulatory support annually in the Unites States. While cardiac transplantation is the preferred treatment for these patients, availability of donors has dedicated when those therapeutic transplantations could occur. In 1990, 2,085 transplants were performed in the United States, while another 1,794 patients awaited transplantation. It has been estimated that from 10 to 40 percent of all heart transplant candidates die while awaiting for donor hearts. The average wait for transplant is currently over ten months. Temporary mechanical support while awaiting donor organs was originally introduced by Cooley and his workers in 1967. Since that time, it has been shown that bridge to transplant is a viable option for patients awaiting a donor heart. Patients surviving the temporary mechanical support have been shown to have a transplant survival similar to that of elective cardiac transplantation patients.[3,4]

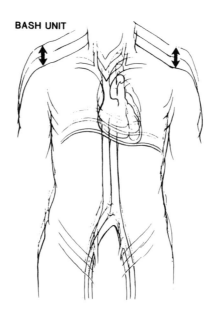

Figure 1. Cardiac assist by synchronized total body acceleration.

This chapter will review the historical development of devices as well as the types of ventricular support systems currently available. It will also present suggestions pertaining to device selection and discuss the expectations, limitations and complications of various methods of mechanical ventricular assist.

HISTORY OF MECHANICAL SUPPORT DEVICES

In 1812, LeGallois stated "...if one could substitute for the heart a kind of injection of arterial blood, either natural or artificially made, one would succeed in maintaining alive indefinitely any part of the body whatsoever".[5] While LeGallois' statement bears proof that the idea was conceptualized much earlier, the actual development of devices of artificially assist circulation was not practical until the discovery of heparin by McLean over 100 years later, in 1916. Lindberg and Carel, in 1930, achieved the first oxygenation of perfused fluid by compressed air. As early as 1934, Debakey described the roller pump which was to be utilized to maintain the continuous transfusion of blood.[6] By 1937, Gibbon had begun his initial work to suggest the therapeutic value of cardiopulmonary bypass in the temporary support of patients with pulmonary emboli. His initial studies of pulmonary artery occlusion in cats supported these early conclusions of the possibilities and potentials of cardiopulmonary bypass.[7,8] In 1944, Dr. Kolff described the first concepts of the membrane oxygenator.[9] As early as 1951, Arntzenius[10] described total body synchronized acceleration for assisting the blood out of the ventricle (Figure 1).

Support of the Failing Heart by Mechanical Devices

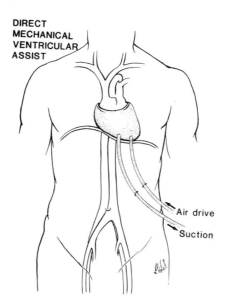

Figure 2. Direct ventricular mechanical assist.

Connolly et al, in 1958, described left heart bypass with left atrium to femoral support for prolonged periods of cross clamping of the aorta.[11] Early disc oxygenators were discovered by Craaford and Bjork in 1948 with bubble oxygenators and veno-venous bypass as early as 1950. In the late 1950's, Anstead et al.[12] suggested direct mechanical compression of the heart to enhance cardiac output (Figure 2).

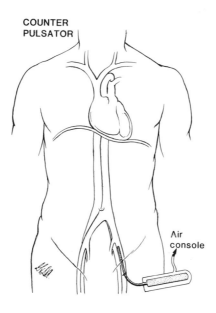

Figure 3. Early form of arterial counterpulsation.

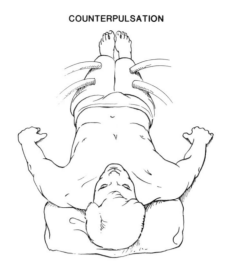

Figure 4. External regional counterpulsation.

In 1960, Kouwenhoven et al. demonstrated that the manual compression of the sternum would support the body during ventricular stand still.[13] This gave birth to the closed chest massage for cardiopulmonary resuscitation and by 1961, Harkins and Bramson, had developed a device capable of external massage by a manual compression of the sternum.[14]

Clauss, in 1961, proposed the concept of counterpulsation as a means of assisted circulation (Figure 3). In part, he drew his conclusions from the

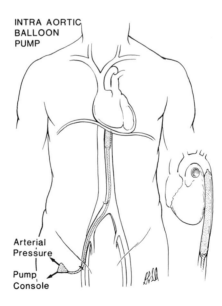

Figure 5. Intra-aortic balloon counterpulsation.

work of Sarnoff and Brahnwald who had previously delineated the relationship of myocardial oxygen consumption to ventricular pressures during the cardiac cycle.[15]

Osbourne first discussed diastolic augmentation by external pulsation pressure in 1962 (Figure 4).

In 1961, Monopoulos and Topaz, while working in the laboratory of William Kolff, first described the concepts of intra-aortic balloon pumping (IABP).[16] This concept was further developed in 1968 by Kantrowitz, who presented excellent clinical results demonstrating the success of IABP in the treatment of cardiogenic shock (Figure 5).[17] In 1970, Birtwell described the use of external body compression for counterpulsation.[18]

It was in 1951 that Dennis actually performed the first cardiopulmonary bypass. While his bypassing techniques were apparently successful, his patient succumbed during the surgery because the presumed atrial septal defect (ASD) to be repaired turned out to be an endocardial cushion defect. Gibbon, is credited with the first successful cardiopulmonary bypass on a human in 1953.[8]

In 1962, Dennis described left heart bypass without thoracotomy achieved with the use of a left atrial cannula introduced from the right jugular vein through the atrial septum.[19] In 1971, Zwart described an ingenious idea of bypassing the left ventricle by inserting a thin walled tube retrograde in the carotid artery in calves and advancing it into the chamber of the left ventricle. Blood was pulled through this cannula and pumped back into the carotid artery with a roller pump to help support the failing left ventricle.[20]

In 1968, Cooley implanted the first artificial heart with a device developed by Liotta. With this device, Cooley supported a patient unable to be weaned from bypass for 64 hours until a donor heart became available.[21] The patient died immediately post transplantation. In 1981, Cooley again used the TAH as a bridge to transplant with similar results.[22] The first successful use of the total artificial heart (TAH) was initiated by the author in 1982 in which the Jarvik 7/100 was implanted in the dentist, Barney Clark. This device supported his life for 112 days until he died of pseudomembranous enterocolitis.[23] During the late 1970's, excellent work on a clinical left ventricular assist device (VAD) was conducted under the direction of John Norman. In his study, 27 patients in cardiogenic shock were supported for varied amounts of times with a pneumatically driven left VAD.[24] Today, VAD for the failing ventricle is a well established therapeutic modality with many devices capable of achieving temporary support.

MECHANICAL SUPPORT DEVICES

Figure 6 demonstrates different types of devices for ventricular support. The ventricles may be directly stimulated by the direct mechanical support (Anstadt cup) or by dynamic cardiomyoplasty.

Both ventricles may be bypassed by pulsatile or nonpulsatile devices or replaced orthotopically by a TAH. The blood may be assisted from within the ventricle chamber by the hemopump or the BASH table.

Aortic counterpulsation with an intra-aortic balloon, dynamic aortic patch, or dynamic muscle pump may assist the failing left ventricle.

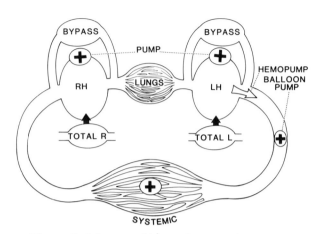

Figure 6. Schemes of types of ventricular support.

Regional external counterpulsation may also lend some temporary circulatory support.

INTRA-AORTIC BALLOON PUMP

Historically, the IABP is the simplest and most commonly used mechanical circulatory assist device with an estimated usage of 70,000 annually in the United States and 30,000 annually internationally. The IABP is a counterpulsating device that is inserted into the descending aorta, either percutaneously, employing a modified Seldinger technique, or through direct cut down onto the femoral artery (Figure 5).

If aorto-iliac disease or previous aorto-iliac grafting precludes cannulation, the device may be placed in the axillary artery, subclavian artery, or even directly into the ascending aorta and advanced antegrade into the descending aorta. In most applications, the device is inserted easily and rapidly by the percutaneous sheath method and can be removed easily at the patient's bedside. Through innovative approaches, the IABP may be used for right heart support by inserting the balloon into a graft surgically attached to the pulmonary artery.

The balloon catheter is a polyurethane, double chambered cannula which fits through a 12 French sheath. Using timed releases of gas, the device console inflates the balloon at the end of the catheter. The timed releases of gas are governed by either the patient's electrocardiogram or by the arterial pressure. The balloon is inflated immediately after closure of the aortic valve displacing 40 cc of blood during diastole into the peripheral and coronary circulations. Previous studies have demonstrated that the IABP may reduce myocardial oxygen consumption in the coronary circulation, decrease heart rate and peak left ventricular systolic wall stress and possibly reduce contractility.[1] Some investigators have suggested that an increase in coronary flow during diastole is brought upon by this type of counterpulsation. The hemodynamic effects of IABP usually demonstrates a 10 to 15 percent decrease in the peak arterial pressure with a 50 to 70 percent increase in the diastolic pressure resulting in a 10 to 20 percent decrease in the left ventricular end-diastolic pressure. Cardiac output in this case may be expected to increase from 10 to 40 percent.

The IABP may be placed for short, as well as intermediate, lengths of time. For short period utilization, anticoagulation is not required. For longer lengths of utilization, the patient may require the addition of anti-platelet drugs. In most clinical applications, the device is used for one to two days; however, the literature cites references to one patient who was supported for 328 days with an IABP and to several patients who were discharged on chronic home balloon pumping.

Since the device is widely available, easily inserted and highly effective when used early, it is the initial device of choice in ventricular support. Intra-aortic balloon support has been successful in its therapeutical use to treat many cases of post cardiotomy cardiac failure, myocardial infarction, cardiogenic shock, pulmonary embolism, cardiomyopathy, and in the treatment of ventricular arrhythmias. In the author's primary hospital for clinical practice, where approximately 1550 open heart procedures and 6000 diagnostic catheterizations were performed in 1992, the IABP was utilized in 108 patients with 41 of these patients expiring (37 percent mortality rate). This degree of mortality has been reported in several other institutions.

Gross aortic insufficiency and acute dissection are absolute contraindications for IABP use. However, prior aortic surgery and aortic aneurysms are only relative contraindications. In presence of sustained, unpredictable arrhythmias, the efficiency of the IABP may be altered due to the difficulty encountered with timing the triggering mechanisms.

The principle complication of the IABP is limb ischemia which presents in approximately 5 to 19 percent of the patients with a 1 percent limb amputation rate. Acute aortic dissection is demonstrated as a complication in approximately 5 percent of the patients. Infection, manifested by either local infection or septicemia, occurs in 3 percent of the patients. Several investigators have estimated a delayed complication of claudication in the extremity where the balloon was inserted to be as high as 48 percent.

This assist device is inexpensive, with the console costing $25,000 to $40,000 and the balloon catheter costing approximately $650 to $750. Advantages of the IABP are that the device is widely available, familiar to most acute care providers, rapidly inserted, and does not require a thoracotomy. The IABP patients are able to be moved around the hospital with relative ease and anticoagulation is not required, enhancing its usefulness in postoperative patients. As a disadvantage, the IABP does not provide total support and except in rare applications, the right heart is not supported.

HEMOPUMP

One of the most innovative methods of temporary cardiac assist is the Hemopump® which was developed by Wampler and is now under investigation by Johnson and Johnson Intervention Systems, Rancho Cordova, CA (Figure 7).

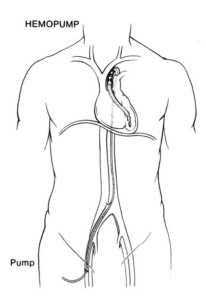

Figure 7. Hemopump®.

This system fills a critical need for a support device in patients where ventricular performance is too profoundly impaired to be resuscitated appropriately with an IABP and may be rapidly inserted without requiring a thoracotomy. This intravascular pump uses the Archimedean screw principle to move the blood from the failing ventricle to the aorta. The pump system consists of a cannula placed into the femoral, iliac or distal aorta and advanced under fluoroscopic control in a retrograde fashion through the aorta and crossing the orifice of the aortic valve with an inlet port placed within the cavity of the left ventricle. The actuator pump is contained within the cylindrical housing and is activated by rotating blades at approximately 2500 rpm. This action draws blood from the left ventricle and moves it within the cylindrical housing and out into the aorta. The rotary motion of the rotating blades is linked inside the catheter by a drive cable and magnetically coupled to a motor inside of a drive console at the bedside of the patient. The inflow, outflow and pumping unit is 25 cm in length and 7 mm (21 French) in diameter with a beveled, flexible tip of silicone rubber. The cannula also contains a purge system which continually lubricates the drive shaft and propeller. After several years of investigation, it has been reported that this will provide relative short termed nonpulsatile flow of approximately 80 percent (3.5 L/min) of the left ventricular output. Until recently, this device was approved for clinical trials in the treatment of cardiogenic shock and as a support for high risk angioplasty under an Investigational Device Exemption (IDE) approved by the Food and Drug Administration (FDA). At present, the FDA has recalled the Hemopump IDE and the device is undergoing further development. However, the Hemopump is currently in use in over 30 centers in Germany, France, Belgium, Holland and England for cardiogenic shock, failure to wean from bypass, high risk percutaneous transluminal coronary angioplasty (PTCA) and bridge to transplant. The device does require moderate anticoagulation. The desired partial thromboplastin time (PTT) is 1.5 to 2.0 times the control value. Obviously, the Hemopump may not be used in patients who have prosthetic aortic valves, known aortic wall disease, known or suspected thoracic or abdominal aortic aneurysm dissections, aortic valve stenosis or insufficiency, or severe aorto-iliac disease. The Hemopump complications have been similar to those of other cardiac assist devices which include vascular injury, thrombus formation, ventricular arrhythmias, bleeding, infection and death. A recent, yet unpublished, multi-institutional study shows that the Hemopump was successfully inserted in 97 patients and resulted in a significant improvement in the hemodynamic status during assistance. In these clinical trial, 42 (27 percent) of the patients survived and the device was removed with the control groups of this study having only a 19 percent survival rate. This device may be an extremely valuable support means in patients with sudden cardiogenic shock in the catheterization laboratory or coronary care unit or in the recovering post cardiotomy patient with low cardiac output.

VENO-ARTERIAL BYPASS WITH PUMP OXYGENATOR

One of the earliest accepted mechanisms of mechanical circulatory assist has been femoral vein to femoral artery bypass using a non-blood primed oxygenator and a pump.[11] This system consists of probably the simplest and least expensive forms of VAD using basic circulatory and devices available to any institution with open heart facilities (Figure 8).

With the advent of Sarns Percar (3M Healthcare, Ann Arbor, MI) or the Bard CPS cardiopulmonary bypass unit (Bard Cardiopulmonary De-

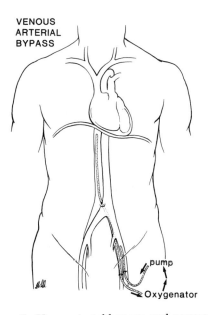

Figure 8. Veno-arterial bypass and oxygenator.

vices, Billerica, MA), the femoral artery can be cannulated through the percutaneous method for arterial access and a long cannula introduced into the vena cava for the venous access. These systems have been developed into portable units for rapid cardiopulmonary bypass for resuscitation in cardiogenic shock and for assisting high risk angioplasties in the catheterization laboratory. These devices consist of a catheter inflow and outflow system, an oxygenator, a heat controller and a centrifugal pump. A roller pump may be used in place of a centrifugal pump. Flows of 4 to 6 L/min are obtained. Patients in cardiogenic shock secondary to myocardial infarction, can be kept alive with this type of support until angiographic studies or angioplasty can be performed, or until the patient can get safely into the operating room and on full routine cardiopulmonary bypass. These devices are used safely for 6 to 7 hours. These portable systems are useful as highly mobile short-term support systems but require regular usage in order to develop and maintain the staffing expertise necessary for rapid, and effective implantation. They are relatively inexpensive with a device console cost of $13,000 to 15,000 and disposable costs of $1,500 per use. Full anticoagulation is required for their use and full time perfusion personnel are needed for device operation.

ECMO

The use of extracorporeal membrane oxygenation (ECMO) in children has been developed since the early 70's and has had considerable experience with its use in patients with respiratory diseases. In children, this type of circuitry involves venous drainage from the right internal jugular vein and arterial reinfusion into the right internal jugular vein and arterial reinfusion into the right carotid artery. A *T*-shaped arterial cannula avoids total occlusion of the carotid artery. This system, however, is generally not suitable for long-term ventricular support mainly due to problems with anticoagulation, hemolysis and infection.[25]

CENTRIFUGAL, ROLLER AND OTHER NONPULSATILE MECHANICAL SUPPORT SYSTEMS

Beyond that of the IABP, the roller or centrifugal pumps have had probably the greatest usage in the world (Figure 9).[3,26,27] Until very recently, the use of these devices for continued mechanical support outside the operating room was not regulated by the FDA. Consequently, patient outcome data with this type of support is likely to have been poorly reported and correlated. While a review of the literature will contain many impressive series, one must remain suspicious that many surgeons who have used these devices may not have reported their poorer results, simply because such reporting and monitoring was not required.

A roller pump or centrifugal pump may be used with various inflow cannulae with blood taken from the right atrium and infused into the pulmonary artery for right heart assist or from the left atrium and infused into the aorta for left heart assist. These devices will generate from 1.5 to 6

Support of the Failing Heart by Mechanical Devices 115

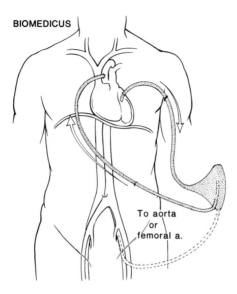

Figure 9. Centrifugal support system.

L/min of nonpulsatile flow. The roller pump, Sarns® impeller, and the Electro-Catheter® systems require full anticoagulation. The Medtronic Biomedicus® moves blood by a series of rotating cones using viscous drag as a propellant.[28] As an advantage, the Biomedicus® pump (Figure 9) requires minimal to no anticoagulation and in actual clinical application, some investigators only anticoagulate the patient during weaning.

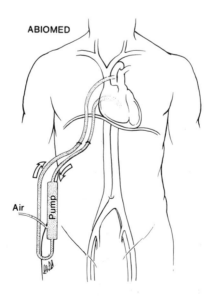

Figure 10. Abiomed® Bus-500.

Because of thrombin accumulation in the pumping chamber, most of the centrifugal pumps' upper limits of duration of support appears to be 5 to 7 days. Pump heads must be changed every 24 to 48 hours. Roller pump systems have the disadvantage of requiring a venous reservoir and have the danger of pumping air if not monitored continuously. These devices have the advantage of being easily available, familiar to all, and until recently, usable without FDA regulation. They are relatively inexpensive, with an average cost of $9,000 to $11,000 for a console and between $150 to $200 for the disposable pump heads. As disadvantages, these devices require constant monitoring by trained personnel and the patients are poorly mobile. These systems carry a significant risk for thromboembolism, infection and hemolysis.

BVS-5000

The BVS-5000 (Abiomed Cardiovascular, Inc., Danvers, MA) is a short-term univentricular or biventricular pulsatile pumping support system (Figure 10).

This is the only system of this type device that is approved by the FDA for general usage. The system consists of single use, pneumatically powered pumping tubes which incorporate an atrial filling chamber and a ventricular pumping chamber. These chambers are comprised of polyurethane bladders. Flow direction is maintained by two polyurethane tri-leaflet valves. The ventricular chamber alternately fills and collapses in response to pulsed gusts of compressed air from the console.[2] Atrial vascular access is achieved with cannulation using a 46 French, wire reinforced cannula. Reinfusion is achieved with cannulation into either the pulmonary artery for right heart assist, or into the ascending aorta for left heart assist, using a flexible cannula attached to a 12 mm woven Dacron graft. The cannulae are usually externalized from the patient's right or left subcostal area, and connected to their respective device chambers. The system maintains a constant stroke volume with monitoring of pump rate and flow rate. This system is fully automated and requires minimal operator input during normal use. The drive system operates on alternate current or can be battery powered. The device is able to produce flow of up to approximately 6.5 L/min. Its use has been reported in over 400 cases worldwide. Fifty-five percent of patients were weaned from the bypass support and 29 percent discharged from the hospital. Worldwide, the device was used 49 percent in post cardiotomy patients, 23 percent in cardiomyopathy patients, 11 percent in acute myocardial infarctions and 11 percent in failed transplant patients. Of the implants, 66 percent were used for biventricular assist, 29 percent left univentricular assist and 4 percent for right univentricular assist (personal communication).

This ventricular assist device represents a useful and practical approach of supporting the heart until myocardial viability is determined. Usually, the heart will declare its ability to recover within 48 to 96 hours. These devices are only moderately expensive, at an approximate cost of $15,000 to $20,000 for the console and approximately $3,000 for the pump. The device requires the specialized training of the support team before hospital usage. Patient mobility is limited with this device.

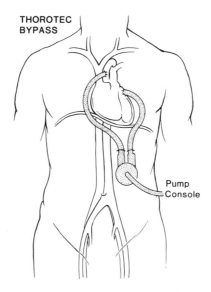

Figure 11. Pierce-Donachy Thoratec VAD.

PIERCE-DONACHY THORATEC® VAD

The Pierce-Donachy Thoratec® VAD (Thoratec Laboratory Corp., Berkeley, CA) consists of a pneumatically pumped ventricle used in a paracorporeal position for either right ventricular or left ventricular support (Figure 11). These ventricles consist of a polyurethane pumping chamber with a 65 mL stroke volume which is pneumatically activated with pulses of alternating positive and negative air pressure. The position of the diaphragm is electronically sensed to allow full 65 mL full-to-empty variable rate system operation.

The pump may also be triggered in an asynchronous or in a synchronous timing pattern. The full-to-empty mode is used in most cases, particularly if the patient is a bridge to transplant candidate.

An advantage of this particular device is that it may be used as a right or left univentricular support mechanism as well as a biventricular support mechanism. Several cannulae are available for outflow connections to the aorta and for atrial or ventricular inflow connectors. Unidirectional flow is obtained through two Bjork Shiley tilting disc valves. Six to 7 L/min of cardiac output may be obtained at 100 beats/min.[29] Various anticoagulation schemes may be used, but usually low-level anticoagulation is used during high pump flow rates. Heparin is used initially in the patient's course and warfarin used later to maintain a prothrombin time (PT) of 1.5 times control. This device is frequently used as a bridge to transplant. Currently, there has been over 255 such implants. Of these, 66 percent of the patients have been transplanted successfully with an overall survival rate of 55 percent. Approximately 69 percent of the implants have been for biventricular support. Most of the usage is for relatively short to moderate time courses. One patient has been maintained for 248 days. This device is still being studied under IDE regulations in the United States but is currently being implanted in over 67 centers and in 11 foreign countries.

With the pumping device placed outside of the body, this allows for a wide range of patient sizes for implantation use. Trouble shooting becomes much easier than with the implanted types of ventricular support. The device is expensive at the approximate cost of $50,000 for the console and approximately $13,000 for the device ventricle. Cardiowest (Tucson, AZ) is also developing a similar pneumatically driven, pulsatile, pumping system yielding promising results.

TCI HEARTMATE®

The Heartmate® blood pump (Thermocardio Systems, Inc., Woburn, MA) is a pulsatile air driven heart which is implanted in the left upper quadrant of the abdomen (Figure 12). The inflow conduit arises from the apex of the left ventricle with the outflow conduit being a flexible cannulae with a Dacron graft sewn onto the ascending aorta. The titanium pump has a flexible polyurethane diaphragm which is bonded to a rigid pusher plate. Pulses of air are delivered from the console to the air chamber immediately behind the pusher plate diaphragm. This action propels blood through the outflow graft into the ascending aorta. Unidirectional flow is achieved by two porcine xenograft valves.[30,31] A unique feature of the Heartmate ventricular assist system is that it incorporates a textured blood surface for all blood contacting surfaces. The textured titanium surface, as well as the textured polyurethane surface, is designed to encourage the formation of pseudo-intima from the blood. Stroke sensors within the pump housing may be used to determine the

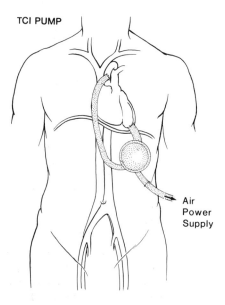

Figure 12. TCI Heartmate® LVAD.

stroke volume and cardiac output and to assist the pump in ejecting its contents when it is 90 percent full (75 mL stroke volume). Synchronization of the pump is also possible from an external QRS detector. Generally, the pump is run by the auto-fill mode to achieve its pulsatile cardiac output. This pump may generate as high as 10 L/min of cardiac output. Adequate anticoagulation can be achieved by using aspirin and dipyridamole after the patient is able to tolerate a diet. Between 1985 and the present, a yet unpublished clinical trial with the pneumatic TCI L-VAD for bridge to transplant includes 134 implants with support ranging from 1 to 324 days. Of these implants, 67 percent of the patients were successfully transplanted with a 59 percent discharge rate from the hospital rate.[32]

A vented electrical system has also been developed by TCI® which consists of the same type of blood surfaces but with an electro-mechanical driver consisting of a low speed torque motor that propels a pusher plate through a pair of helical cams. This system has the potential of being fully implanted and should be an excellent device for chronic support of the failed left ventricle.

This device has the disadvantage of being able to support only the left ventricle. Between 1991 and 1992, four patients with idiopathic cardiomyopathy underwent implantation of the electric Heartmate® L-VAD with excellent long-term support and excellent mobility of the patient. This device also requires an IDE. TCI Heartmate® Systems are expensive but have excellent long-term supporting results.

NOVACOR®

The Novacor® pump (Baxter Health Care Corp., Oakland, CA) is a pulsatile left ventricular assist device (Figure 13). The Novacor pump was

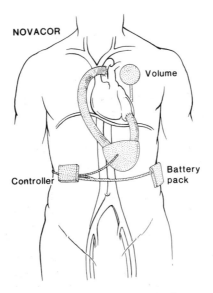

Figure 13. Novacor® LVAD.

designed as an electrically driven, potentially fully implantable, left VAD to be used for chronic cardiac support.[33] The pump consists of a seamless polyurethane sack which is bonded to symmetrically opposed pusher plates and a housing that incorporates valve fittings. The pump uses pericardial valves and is encapsulated in a fiber glass reinforced shell. The pump weights approximately 3.3 kg and occupies a volume of 400 mL. The device is positioned in the left upper quadrant of the anterior abdominal wall and the inflow conduit is cannulated to the left ventricular apex with the outflow conduit anastomosed to the ascending aorta. The pusher plates are powered by a solenoid that converts electrical energy from the control console to power the compression of the blood sack. The pump is linked to the console by a power line and vent which exit the skin in the right lower abdominal quadrant.

Transducer signals provide information concerning filling volumes, pump output, and pump rate. The pump has a nominal stroke volume of 70 mL and can pump in excess of 8 L/min. This pump may be triggered by timing of the EKG for a synchronous mode, from changes in the rate of pump filling, or at a fixed rate setting. Initially, the patient requires continuous anticoagulation heparin infusion to maintain a PTT of 1.5 times the control and later is switched to warfarin therapy (PT of 20 to 30 percent of the control value).

Clinical investigations started in 1984 enrolled 126 of these implants; 74 (59 percent) patients have been successfully transplanted with the longest post transplant survival of 8 years. The Novacor® has been used for support times ranging from 1 to 370 days. Some patients were able to live outside of the hospital while undergoing support. This device is currently being modified to become a fully implanted device requiring no percutaneous connections.

The device is only capable of producing left ventricular support; therefore, its use in biventricular failure may be limited. Furthermore, the patients must weigh at least 50 kg and currently be designated as candidates for transplantation. An IDE is required for it use. Each pumping device cost approximately $24,000 with an approximate cost of $65,000 for the console.

ORTHOTOPIC BIVENTRICULAR REPLACEMENT PROSTHESIS (ARTIFICIAL HEART)

The Symbion Total Artificial Heart® is a pneumatically driven device that consists of two separate ventricles, one replacing the left ventricle and one replacing the right ventricle (Figure 14). This device is placed in an orthotopic position after excising the natural failed ventricles while retaining the capacitant atrial chambers. Unidirectional flow is obtained in each ventricle by two Medtronic-Hall® (Medtronic, Inc., Minneapolis, MN) mechanical prosthetic valves.[34] The Symbion Artificial Heart® has two basic models, a 70 mL stroke volume design and a larger model with a stroke volume of 100 mL for use in larger patients (greater than 80 kg). The ventricles are made of layered polyurethane with a diaphragm activated by pulsed, positive air pressure through two drive lines exiting in the left upper

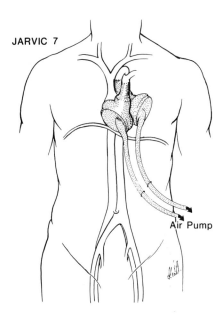

Figure 14. Symbion® Jarvik 7 orthotopic ventricular replacement "Total Artificial Heart".

quadrant of the abdomen. The drive console maintains the positive pulses of air pressure. Measurement of the velocity of the vented air returning to atmosphere is used to determine the cardiac output and filling characteristics of the ventricles. The heart may be adjusted to variable heart rates as well as to duration of systole and diastole.[35]

The Symbion Artificial Heart® is no longer available through an IDE, but a quite similar device is now available through a revised IDE by Cardiowest, Inc., Tuscon, AZ. The heart will respond to a Starling, regulated curve with stroke volume being directly proportional to the atrial pressures filling the ventricles. As a bridge to transplant, the Symbion Artificial Heart® has been used in 185 patients and has approximately a 65 percent successful transplantation rate. Approximately 50 percent of the post transplantation patients were discharged from the hospital.[4] The time period for supporting circulation with the Symbion Total Artificial Heart® for bridge to transplant ranges from 1 to 603 days with usual transplantation within the first three days.

Five patients have received the Symbion Artificial Heart as a permanent device. The range of implantation times to death on these patients range from 10 to 620 days. This device is well suited for complete replacement of totally irreversible ventricular failure in patients awaiting definitive transplantation. Some investigators have asserted that there is a higher prosthetic infection rate in this device as compared to the paracorporeal pump when used for bridge to transplant.[36] As the Symbion Artificial Heart® required in-house sterilization within each participating facility, monitoring for preparatory sterilization was without a given control group and device infection rates varied widely between centers.

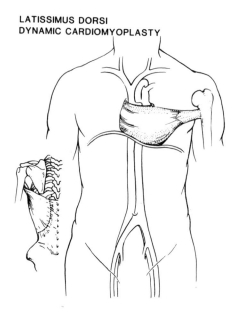

Figure 15. Dynamic Cardiomyoplasty.

DYNAMIC CARDIOMYOPLASTY

The use of the autogenous skeletal muscle for support to the failing ventricle represents a new approach to direct cardiac assist (Figure 15).

At present, the best clinical results have been achieved by using the left latissimus dorsi as a muscle wrap around the failing ventricle. Electrical stimulation of the skeletal muscle is usually initiated several weeks after the operation with progressive muscle conditioning protocols.[37] In the literature, over 120 cardiomyoplasty procedures have been performed worldwide with a generalized improvement in NYHA functional class and exercise performance in patients with refractory heart failure. Progressive sequential stimulation generally requires over a six week course to fully condition the muscle for maximum support. This system has an advantage of using the patient's own tissue for support and does not require any anticoagulation or implanted material except for the small pacemaker inserted for muscle stimulation. The disadvantage of this therapy is that complete cardiac support cannot be obtained and the full efficacy of support may, at many times, require several months for actualization. Measurable hemodynamic improvement many times does not equal that of the functional improvement in the patient.[37,38] Several explanations have been presented for this enhanced functional improvement. One is the actual active component from the transformed muscle. It has also been postulated that the muscle wrap may stabilize the ventricular dilatation which occurs during further decompensation of the heart muscle.

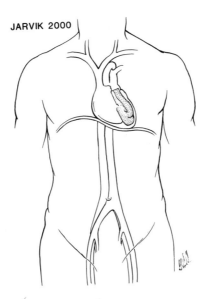

Figure 16. Jarvik 2000.

Future devices

Several future devices using impeller type electrical turbines are being currently developed. A prototype of this device is the Jarvik 2000 which is placed in the cavity of the failing left ventricle. The impeller assists blood from the left atrium into the aorta (Figure 16).

DIRECT MECHANICAL VENTRICULAR ACTUALIZATION

This method employs an elliptical contoured cup which fits over the right and left ventricles. It is held in place by a vacuum source sustaining a constant negative pressure (Figure 2). Pulse pressure is generated through to a flexible silastic diaphragm which represents the actual pumping chambers. The pump can be implanted rapidly onto the heart through a left thoracotomy. The positive and negative pneumatic forces are generated from an external console. The continuing massaging action of the pump is controlled from the pneumatic drive system. This device is capable of producing cardiac outputs of 80 to 110 percent of control. It has the advantage of being rapidly implanted, (in some cases less than two minutes), and requires no anticoagulation. It is generally used for a relatively short time assistance, however there is one case reported of over 56 hours of circulatory support until a successful cardiac transplantation was possible.[39]

SELECTION OF VENTRICULAR ASSIST DEVICES

There are many considerations in the selection of a ventricular support device. The nature of the physiological defect must be determined.

If ventricular failure is predominantly left-sided, then one device may be chosen over the other. IABP and Hemopumps® support left ventricular failure. At the current time, the Novacor® and TCI Heartmate® are available for isolated left-sided failure only. If right-sided failure should occur during the course of these devices, other support systems such as pulmonary artery counterpulsation, centrifugal support pumps, Cardiowest®, or Thoratec® devices may be added for right ventricular support.

Although many of the paracorporeal devices purport to be able to support the entire cardiac output during ventricular fibrillation, most of the devices, whether centrifugal or pulsatile, do not handle this hemodynamic situation as well as advertised. TAH may be required for support in these types of patients.

Considerations of reversibility should determine the nature of the support. In patients with end-stage dilated left ventricular myocardiopathy or scarred fibrotic left ventricular aneurysm, or other end-stage situation, reversibility may not be a factor. In these cases, the pumps involving left ventricular apex withdrawal systems such as TCI®, Thoratec®, or Novacor® may provide excellent pumping mechanics without concern of removing potentially recoverable left ventricular muscle. If the patient is believed to have a reversible situation, left ventricular apical pumping is probably not the most desirable form of cannulation. In a similar manner, patients with devices used for bridge to transplant, may be pumped at fixed rate or nonsynchronously pumping since the hemodynamics of the coronary perfusion may not have to be considered. If, however, the injured myocardium is believed to be recoverable, then counterpulsation pumping may be desirable.

The size of the patient is critical in determination of the type of pumps used. In children, ECMO may be the only alternative for the temporary support. In small patients, the external pumps from Cardiowest®, Thoratec®, or the centrifugal pumps may be the only devices available. In larger size men, the Novacor®, TCI®, and TAH may be implanted.

Sudden ventricular failure occurring in the catheterization laboratory may be only amenable to the IABP, mobile veno-arterial systems or the Hemopump systems in order to stabilize the patient. In the cases of complete cardiac arrest that is not responsive to cardiopulmonary resuscitation, the placement of these devices is very difficult even with an experienced team. Mobilization of the patient and rapid open heart surgery may yield better results in this group of patients.

Post cardiotomy bypass failure is, in most cases, believed to be reversible. A centrifugal pump or pneumatic bypass with cannulation in the

Table 1. Indications for Post Cardiotomy Ventricular Support.

Fully surgically corrected anatomical defect
Satisfactory volume status
Full inotropic or vasodilator support
Corrected metabolic parameters
Intra-aortic balloon pump
Less than four hours bypass

Table 2. Hemodynamic Guidelines for VAD Placement*

Cardiac Index	<1.8 L/min/m^2
Systolic Blood Pressure	<90 mmHg
Left or Right Atrial Pressure	>20 mmHg
Urine Output	<20 mL/min
Systemic Vascular Resistance	>21 dynes·sec/cm^5

*Despite adequate preload and maximal pharmacological support and intra-aortic balloon pump.

Table 3. Criteria for Isolated Left Ventricular Support.

Left Atrial Pressure	>20 mmHg
Mean Pulmonary Artery Pressure	<15 mmHg
No Arrhythmias	
Near Normal Right Ventricular Function	

atrium such as the Thoratec®, Cardiowest® or Abiomed® devices may be used as support measures.

The length of time of support needed must be considered. In most cases, if myocardial recovery in post cardiotomy patients is expected, it will generally manifest itself within the first 24 to 72 hours. This time course is easily handled by the Abiomed® centrifugal pumps, Thoratec® or Cardiowest® devices. If, however, longer support is necessary and the patient is a candidate for bridge to transplant, systems such as the Thoratec®, the Novacor®, or the Cardiowest TAH® or VAD should be used because these are more successful bridging pumps and will allow the patient more mobility.

Almost all of the devices covered are under IDE approval with the FDA. While the Thoratec®, Novacor®, TCI Heartmate®, Hemopump®, Cardiowest® pumps and the dynamic cardiomyoplasty may appear to be very attractive, one must not loose track of the fact that these systems require FDA approval for participation. Extensive team building, rigid scientific protocol and expensive training periods as well as required back up in inventory of devices must be met. Institutions may encounter $200,000 to $300,000 in start up costs for these requirements. The only FDA approved device for ventricular support at this time is the Abiomed®. This device also requires a training period that may incur expense. Presently, FDA is considering the regulation of the centrifugal pumps which may impact on the ability of a surgeon to use these devices outside of the

Table 4. Criteria for Isolated Right Ventricular Support.

Right Atrial Pressure	>20 mmHg
Left Atrial Pressure	<20 mmHg
No Arrhythmias	
Near Normal Left Ventricular Function	

Table 5. Criteria for Bi-Ventricular Support.

Left & Right Atrial Pressures	>20 mmHg
Ventricular Tachycardia or Fibrillation	
Severely impaired right and left ventricular function (echocardiography, catheterization, or MUGA scan)	

operating room. The impact of the regulation of usage of this type of common device may have an impact on the industrial supplier, institution, and surgeon. As a practical matter, the surgeon who is familiar with IABP, and the available Abiomed® device will cover their patient's needs of acute use well. If the institution has a transplantation program, there is a need for one of the longer support systems and FDA approval of one of these systems should be sought. It is hopeful that within the next several years, many of these restricted pumps will become available for general use.

Several investigators have suggested that non-pulsatile pumping may not provide adequate needs for the body's perfusion requirements. These reports present the isolated renal function during various perfusion modes.[40,41] While the definitive answer has not been found yet, others have reported that end organ function may be preserved in patients with a centrifugal pump in place by placing an IABP for pulsation.[33]

GENERALIZED PRINCIPLES OF MECHANICAL VENTRICULAR SUPPORT

Of paramount importance in establishing a ventricular support system within an institution is the intense, complete preparation of protocols to direct each aspect of the clinical course. Before embarking on this form of treatment, the physician must have an unwavering commitment from the medical and nursing staff, the institution, and from the company sponsoring the device. The outcomes of these devices are directly and proportionally related to the clinical readiness and experience of the surgical and medical teams. There is no question that the FDA, in requiring clinical readiness for IDE approval, has insured the safety of patients by mandating the presence of a high degree of clinical proficiency and training before allowing the experimental usages of many of these devices.

One of the most important discerning factors in the outcome success of these devices to determine patient salvage is the appropriateness of patient selection and the matching of the devices used to the needs of the clinical situation encountered. Many of these decisions can be made more easily and with a greater degree of deliberation by the establishment of clinical directive protocols before the actual need arises. As the early history of the usage of IABP suggested, the success of this device was directly related to how rapidly and early in the course of ventricular failure the device was inserted. Decisions to initiate ventricular support must be made rapidly with great emphasis placed on discerning the viability of the myocardium and the end organs prior to devices implantation. Clinical protocols addressing postoperative care must be established preoperatively. These protocols need to direct anticoagulation regimens and to outline the treatment of postoperative complications, including infection, neurological sequelae, and renal insufficiency.

The importance of an active transplantation program or mobilization plans should be made before the selection of the patient is undertaken. Most transplant teams should have a usable device in place because of the relatively frequent need for bridge to transplant. Several investigators have estimated a ventricular device requirement in 0.2 to 1.0 percent of post cardiotomy patients.

Before the actual device is selected, patient considerations of age, weight, overall medical condition and social support structure, must be weighed to determine the patient candidacy for transplantation.

Considerations of the degree of pulmonary hypertension and the presence of other pre-existing physiological problems, such as insulin-dependent diabetes, COPD, history of peripheral or cerebral vascular disease, active infection, or malignancies must be addressed. The patient must have no evidence of blood dyscrasia or peptic ulcer disease because of the need for anticoagulation. The body habitus must be carefully evaluated against the limitation restraints of each device. A well selected patient, rapidly diagnosed and treated appropriately will have a good outcome. The converse is also true.

In surgical patients unable to be weaned from cardiopulmonary bypass, the patient must have had a technically satisfactory operation. If bypass weaning is being handicapped by poor valve function, this problem must be evaluated for its potential for surgical intervention and repaired as indicated. Any incomplete revascularizations must be corrected in order to give the patient maximum recovery benefits. If the patient has had a technically satisfactory operation and still does not wean, an intraoperative assessment of the patient's chances of ventricular recovery should be made. VADs can never be a substitute for poor surgical intervention. The patient who is believed to have the potential for myocardial recovery, should then be treated with inotropic and vasodilation drugs with careful intraoperative monitoring of adequate volume loading. IABP should be rapidly instituted at this time. Many patients may benefit by simply returning to cardiopulmonary bypass in this period to rest the failing ventricle; however, the importance of rapid decisions before the patient's ventricles and end organs are irreversibly compromised is critical. Many authors suggest that if the patient has had over 4 hours of bypass time, the chances of successful outcome are grim.

General criteria for VAD placement vary but guidelines suggest that a patient with a cardiac index under 1.8 L/min with left atrial pressures greater than 20 mm in the view of optimal volume status, maximal inotropic support, correction of metabolic deficits, and IABP would be a candidate for ventricular assist.

The situation, at that point, should entail choices of devices and the need for right ventricular support. Pure left ventricular support may be useful if the left atrial pressure is greater than 20 mmHg and mean pulmonary artery pressure is under 15 mmHg with normal pulmonary vascular resistance, no arrhythmias, and no evidence of right ventricular failure.

Table 6. Overall Results - All Years ASAIO - ISHLT Registry { }

Indication	No. of Patients	Weaned or Transplanted (%)	Discharged (%)
PCCS	1223	45.1	24.7
Bridge to Transplant	550	67.6	45.3
AMI	85	29.4	12.9
TOTAL:	1858	51.1	30.2

PCCS = Postcardiotomy cardiac support; AMI = Acute myocardial infarction

If, however, the right atrial pressure is greater than 20 mmHg and no arrhythmias and normal left ventricular function, a right ventricular device alone may be required.

If the left and right atrial pressures are both over 20 mmHg, or if there is ventricular fibrillation, tachycardia, or other malignant arrhythmias or severely impaired ventricular function evidenced preoperatively by echocardiogram, catheterization, or multi-gated acquisition (MUGA) scan, the surgeon should immediately proceed with full biventricular support.

The decisions of whether to support the patient with univentricular or biventricular pumping is controversial. Of the patients who have received left ventricular support only, 25 percent will have to return to the operating room for supplemented right ventricular support.

Investigators have postulated that the complete unloading of the left ventricle impairs septal movement which interferes with right ventricular output.[42,43] In patients with left ventricular support only, treatment of 24 to 48 hours with inotropic and volume support may be sufficient to relieve the initial stunned right ventricle.

Some investigators suggest the rapid institution of biventricular support for right sided-failure adds very little to the complication rate of left-sided support only. However, most outcome data show that biventricular support carries a worse outcome. These data can be misleading and may simply illustrate the clinical course of the more morbid patients who are straight forth candidates for biventricular support.

COMPLICATIONS OF VENTRICULAR ASSIST DEVICES

A review of the combined complications in the American Society of Artificial Internal Organs-International Society of Heart Lung Transplant (ASAIO-ISHLT) registry demonstrates that 44 to 57 percent of the patients suffer bleeding complications, approximately 25 percent renal failure, 20 percent respiratory failure, 12 to 14 percent infection and neurological complications of 10 percent in the post pericardiotomy and bridge to transplant groups but over 18 percent in the acute myocardial infarction groups. Mechanical failure of the devices represents only 2 to 5 percent.[3]

Bleeding Complications

Since many of these patients have undergone a period of metabolic instability during the resuscitation as well as a prolonged cardiopulmonary bypass, bleeding complications would be well expected. These devices also have large surfaces in contact with blood, consumption of coagulation factors as a result of contact activation may also result in bleeding tendencies.[44-46] Most of the cannulas for inflow and outflow are attached to active cardiac muscle in motion in which spreading of suture lines is also a common source of bleeding. Most of the patient's heparin is fully reversed post bypass with protamine. There should be a fine balance between anticoagulation to prevent embolic phenomena from activation of clotting factors and a postoperative bleeding event.

All patients require hemostatic resuscitation during surgery with great emphasis on the replacement of platelets and coagulation factors. Rapid early evacuation and re-exploration for bleeding is critical with the institution of fibrin glue and other local hemostatic materials at the sites of cannulation. The diagnosis of tamponade in these devices is difficult as the symptoms of ventricular failure frequently mask the development of underlying tamponade. Tamponade also may present itself as a late device implant complication. The use of transesophageal echocardiography (TEE) has improved a great deal in the diagnosis of tamponade.[47]

Thromboembolism

Since all devices have been known to activate clotting, thromboembolism with the occurrence of neurological complications, from TIA's to stroke, is common to all of these devices. Strict anticoagulation protocols must be followed and constantly updated to meet the changing clinical situations. Most investigators suggest treatment with low molecular weight dextran at approximately 25 mL/min and dipyridamole 100 mg every 6 hours through the nasal gastric tube after the initial postoperative bleeding stops. At this time, a continuous heparin drip to maintain PTT in the range of 50 to 60 sec is instituted until the patient is able to absorb through the gastrointestinal tract at which time warfarin is started to maintain PT of 16 to 20 sec. During periods of low pump output such as weaning, additional levels of anticoagulation may be used for prevention of thromboembolism.[44,46,48,49]

Infection

Many of these patients are immunologically suppressed[49] from the chronic disease as well as from resuscitative events. Additionally, they are at greater risk of infection because of multi-organ failure and because they require prolonged intravenous and arterial monitoring lines.[50] Pneumonias are a constant source of problem particularly with prolonged respiratory support. Presently, most of the cardiac assist devices have percutaneous lines which may be sites of ascending infection. The seeding of the devices may not be as much due to the percutaneous lines as vascular seeding from many other sites.[51,52] Strict care and handling of all percutaneous sites as well as removal of all possible sources of infection is important.[36,51,53]

Renal failure

Many of these patients develop acute tubular necrosis for various reasons from low flow periods, resuscitative events, metabolic defects, and high transfusion requirements. Acute tubular necrosis, while adds an increased morbidity, generally is reversed with aggressive hemodialysis, ultrafiltration or peritoneal dialysis.

Hemolysis

Hemolysis is frequently observed during the early course of the devices, however, the normal removal of the freed hemoglobin is well tolerated by the patient. This may be, however, at a risk of overloading the reticuloendothelial system and decrease the ability of the immune system to fight infection. Active research is now being pursued to develop new pumps that are gentler to the blood.

RESULTS OF THE MECHANICAL VENTRICULAR ASSIST PUMPS AND THE TOTAL ARTIFICIAL HEART

Over the past several years, the ASAIO and the ISHLT have established a registry of ventricular assist pump results.[3] This voluntary registry has combined overall results of over 1,858 mechanical ventricular assist pumps. Table 6 shows the overall indications and the success of the devices.

A review of these data demonstrates that the best overall outcome is in bridge to transplant patients. In these cases, the decision to bridge the patient was usually made before surgical intervention in patients who readily fit transplantation protocols. Many of these patients did not undergo severe resuscitative measures or prolonged pump times as the post pericardiotomy or the acute myocardial infarctions patients. The bridge to transplant group was approximately 10 years younger in age than the other groups. The type of devices used between the three groups were also slightly different; of the patients undergoing left ventricular support as bridge to transplant, 47 percent of pumps used were pneumatic, 35 percent were electric and 18 percent were centrifugal pumps. These various devices demonstrated a 69 to 78 percent overall transplantation rate with 77 to 94 percent of the patients being discharged post-transplant. The TAH (190 patients) as bridge to transplant, had a 71 percent transplantation rate, however, only 50 percent of the transplanted patients were discharged. The best bridge to transplant results were with the isolated left ventricular assist (183 patients) of which 73 percent were transplanted and 89 percent of the transplanted patients were actually discharged from the hospital. The acute myocardial infarction group results demonstrate 61 percent predominance of left ventricular assist devices and 38 percent usage of biventricular assist devices. Twelve percent of the patients were weaned from their biventricular devices and 38.5 percent weaned from left ventricular assist devices.

The discharge values showed a 17.3 percent discharge of the left ventricular assist group and only a 6.3 percent discharge rate from the biventricular assist devices. The combined registry of post cardiotomy shock patients showed that 71 percent of the patients were sustained with centrifugal pumps and only 27 percent with pneumatic pumps. Both types of pumps had 45 to 46 percent of patients weaned and approximately 25 percent discharged. Fifty-five percent of the pneumatic pumps used were left ventricular only, whereas 34 percent were biventricular and 8 percent were right ventricular. Only 34 percent of the biventricular devices patients were weaned as opposed to 51 percent of the patients using the left ventricular device. The clinical registry also demonstrated that the post pericardiotomy syndrome patients were supported for an average of 3.8 days while the bridge to transplant's mean length of support was over 24 days. Acute myocardial infarction patients were supported for a mean of 5.6 days.

HEALTH CARE REFORM AND ETHICAL DILEMMA

With current mandates for health care reform and their encompassing cost containment requisites for patient care, constant analysis is being required for use of the assistive devices. Questions of the cost effectiveness of many of these expensive devices of seemingly low yield salvage are surfacing in the clinical setting as well as in the media. The common theme in most reform movements is change in the focus of health care delivery. The focus moves toward health maintenance and preventative health care measures. Institutions face, and will continue to face, difficult decisions on the continuation of programs such as heart transplantation and programs that incur expensive, prolonged life-support systems. These programs will be in competition for funding with programs that promulgate the new focus of health care, i.e., programs that will foster a higher yield in long-term cost savings and meet the direct needs of a larger population.

The once proverbial constant of saving a life without regard to cost is a passing reflection of an altruistic society that is now looking for a change and solutions. These changing factors place important emphasis on thoughtful patient selection with devices fitted appropriately to the institution and patient's needs. Meticulously conducted scientific studies with accurate registry of all patient outcomes and the frank, open deliberation of benefits are imperative to the survival of research in the area of assistive devices.

Difficult ethical decisions of support versus no support and imminent death must be made at appropriate clinical times. Poor clinical outcomes and impending hopeless situations should not be the precipitating forces for the use of assistive devices. The importance of pre-device planning and accurate patient selection cannot be stressed enough. Last ditch approaches to prolonging life can obscure the scientific merits and efficacy of devices and may add doom to their continued research.

It is touted throughout health care reform that the roles of health care providers will change and that new focuses for delivery will emerge. Let us stand committed that the roles of patient advocate and promoter of medical research will remain *unchanged*, and that the focus for decreased morbidity and mortality for cardiac patients will remain foremost in all of our goals.

REFERENCES

1. Bregman D: Mechanical support of the failing heart. Curr Prob Surg 1976;13:1.
2. Guyton RA, Schonberger AM, Everts PAM, et al: Postcardiotomy shock: Clinical evaluation of the BVS 5000 biventricular support system. Ann Thorac Surg 1993;56:346-356.
3. Pae WE Jr: Ventricular assist devices and total artificial hearts: A combined registry experience. Ann Thorac Surg 1993;55(1):295-298.
4. Joyce LD, Johnson KE, Pierce WS, DeVries WC, Semb BK, Copeland JG, Griffith BP, Cooley DA, Frazier OH, Cabrol C, et al: Summary of the world experience with clinical use of total artificial hearts as heart support devices. J Heart Transplant 1986;5(3):229-35.
5. LeGallois JJC: Experiences sur le principe de la vie. Notamment sur celui des movements du coeur, et sur le siege de ce principe; suivies du rapport fait a la premiere classe de l'institute sur celles relatives aux movemens due coeur. Paris, D'Hautel, 1912.
6. DeBakey ME: Left ventricular bypass pump for cardiac assistance. Clinical experience. Am J Cardiol 1971;27:3.
7. Gibbon JH Jr: Artificial maintenance of circulation during experimental occlusion of pulmonary artery. Arch Surg 1937;34:1105.
8. Gibbon JH Jr: Application of a mechanical heart and lung apparatus to cardiac surgery. Minn Med 1954;37:171.
9. Kolff WJ, Effler DB, Groves LK, Peereboom G, Moraca PP: Disposable membrane oxygenator (heart-lung) machine and its use in experimental surgery. Cleveland Clin Q 1956;23:69.
10. Arntzenius AC: Discussion of Ware RW, et al: Inertial cardiac assistance. Trans Am Soc Artif Intern Organs 1971;17:219.
11. Connolly JE, Becaner MB, Bruns DL, Lowenstein JM, Storli E: Mechanical support of the circulation in acute heart failure. Surgery 1958;44:255.
12. Anstadt GL, Blakemore W, Baue A: A new instrument for prolonged mechanical cardiac massage. Circulation 1965;(Suppl)32:43.
13. Kouwenhoven WB, Jude JR, Knickerbocker GG: Closed-chest cardiac massage. JAMA 1960;173:1064.
14. Harkins G, Bramson ML: Mechanical external cardiac massage for cardiac arrest and for support of the failing heart. A preliminary communication. Surg Res 1961;1:197.
15. Clauss RH, Birtwell WC, Albertal G, Lunzer S, Taylor WJ, Fosberg AM, Harken DE: Assisted circulation. I. The arterial counterpulsator. J Thorac Cardiovasc Surg 1961;41:447.
16. Monopoulos SD, Topaz S, Kolff W: Diastolic balloon pumping (with carbon dioxide) in the aorta - a mechanical assitance to the failing circulation. Am Heart J 1962;63:669.
17. Kantrowitz A, Tjonneland S, Freed PS, Phillips SJ, Butner AN, Sherman JC: Initial clinical experience with intraaortic balloon pumping in cardiogenic shock. JAMA 1968;203:113-118.
18. Birtwell WC, Giron F, Ruiz U, Norton RL, Soroff HS: The regional hemodynamic response to synchronous external pressure assist. Trans Am Soc Artif Organs 1970;16:462.
19. Dennis C, Carlens E, Senning A, Hall DP, Moreno JR, Capelletti RR, Wesolowski SA: Clinical use of a cannula for left heart bypass without thoracotomy. Ann Surg 1962;156:623.
20. Zwart HHJ, Kralios AC, Kwan-Gett CS, Backman DK, Foote JL, Andrade JD, Kolff WJ: Transarterial closed-chest left ventricular bypass for desperate heart failure. Adv Cardiol 1971;6:157.
21. Cooley DA, Lidotta D, Hallman GL: Orthotopic cardiac prosthesis for two-staged cardiac replacement. Am J Cardiol 1969;24:730.
22. Cooley DA, Akutsu T, Norman JC, Serrato MA, Frazier OH: Total artificial heart in two-staged cardiac transplantation. Cardiovasc Dis Bull Texas Heart Institute 1981;8:305.
23. DeVries WC, Anderson JL, Joyce LD, Anderson FL, Hammond EH, Jarvik RK, Kolff WJ: Clinical use of the total artificial heart. N Engl J Med 1984;310(5):273-8.
24. Norman JC, Fuqua JM, Bennett GG, Trono R, Hibbs CVR, Edmonds CH, Igo SR, Cooley DA: An intracorporeal (abdominal) left ventricular assist device: Initial clinical trials. Arch Surg 1977;112:1442.

25. Golding LA, Crouch RD, Stewart RW, Novoa R, Lytle BW, McCarthy PM, Taylor PC, Loop FD, Cosgrove DM 3d: Postcardiotomy centrifugal mechanical ventricular support. Ann Thorac Surg 1992;54(6):1059–1063.
26. Pennington DG, Swartz MT: Circulatory support in infants and children. Ann Thorac Surg 1993;55(1):233–237.
27. Magovern GJ Jr: The biopump and postoperative circulatory support. Ann Thorac Surg 1993;55(1):245–249.
28. Killen DA, Piehler JM, Borkon AM, et al: Bio-medicus ventricular assist device for salvage of cardiac surgical patients. Ann Thorac Surg 1991;52:230–235.
29. Farrar DJ, Hill JD: Univentricular and biventricular throratec VAD support as a bridge to transplantation. Ann Thorac Surg 1993;55(1):276–282.
30. Frazier OH: Thermo cardiosystems left ventricular assist device (Letter). Ann Thorac Surg 1992;54(5):1019–1020.
31. Frazier OH: Chronic left ventricular support with a vented electric assist device. Ann Thorac Surg 1993;55(1):273–275.
32. Abou-Awdi NL, Frazier OH: The HeartMate: A left ventricular assist device as a Bridge to Cardiac Transplantation. Transplant Proceedings 1992;24(5):2002–2003.
33. Portner PM, Baumgartner WA, Cabrol C, Frazier OH: Internal pulsatile circulatory support. Ann Thorac Surg 1993;55(1):261–265.
34. DeVries WC, Joyce LD: The artificial heart. CIBA Clinical Symposia 1983;35(6):1–32.
35. DeVries WC: Surgical technique for implantation of the Jarvik-7-100 total artificial heart. JAMA 1988;259(6):875–80.
36. Griffith BP, Kormos RL, Hardesty RL, et al: The artificial heart: Infection related morbidity and its effect on transplantation. Ann Thorac Surg 1988;45:409.
37. Carpentier A, Chachques JC, Acar C, et al: Dynamic cardiomyoplasty at seven years. J Thorac Cardiovasc Surg 1993;106(1):42–53.
38. Bocchi EA, Moreira LFP, deMoraes AV, et al: Effects of dynamic cardiomyoplasty on regional wall motion, ejection fraction, and geometry of left ventricle. Circulation 1992(Suppl. II)86(5):231–235.
39. Lowe JE, Anstadt MP, Van Trigt P, et al: First successful bridge to cardiac transplantation using direct mechanical ventricular actuation. Ann Thorac Surg 1991;52:1237–1245.
40. German JC, Chalmers GS, Hirai J, Mukherjee ND, Wakabayashi A, Connolly JE: Comparison of nonpulsatile and pulsatile extracorporeal circulation on renal tissue perfusion. Chest 1972;61:65.
41. Many M, Giron F, Birtwell WC, Deterling RA, Soroff HS: Effects of depulsation of renal blood flow upon renal function and renin secretion. Surg 1969;66:242.
42. Kawai A, Kormos RL, Mandarino WA, Morita S, Deneault LG, Gasior TA, Armitage JM, Griffith BP: Differential regional function of the right ventricle during the use of a left ventricular assist device. ASAIO J 1992;38(3):M676–678.
43. Chow E, Brown CD, Farrar DJ: Effects of left ventricular pressure unloading during LVAD support on right ventricular contractility. ASAIO J 1992;38(3):M473–476.
44. Copeland JG 3d, Frazier HO, McBride LR, Turina MI, Cabrol C: Circulatory Support 1991. The Second International Conference on Circulatory Support for Severe Cardiac Failure. Anticoagulation. Ann Thorac Surg 1993;55(1):213–216.
45. Copeland JG, Harker LA, Joist JH, DeVries WC: Circulatory support 1988: Bleeding and anticoagulation. Ann Thorac Surg 1989;47(1):87–95.
46. Levinson MM, Smith RG, Cork RC, et al: Thromboembolic complications of the Jarvik-7 total artificial heart: case report. Artif Organs 1986;10:236–244.
47. Barzilai B, Davila-Roman VG, Eaton MH, Rosenbloom M, Spray TL, Wareing TH, Cox JL, Kouchoukos NT: Transesophageal echocardiography predicts successful withdrawal of ventricular assist devices. J Thorac Cardiovasc Surg 1992;104(5):1410–1416.
48. Didisheim P, Olsen DB, Farrar DJ, et al: Infections and thromboembolism with implantable cardiovascular devices. ASAIO Trans 1989;35:54–70.
49. Ward RA, Wellhausen SR, Dobbins JJ, Johnson GS, DeVries WC: Thromboembolic and infectious complications of total artificial heart implantation. Ann NY Acad Sciences 1987;516:638–50.

50. Hill JD, Griffith BP, Meli M, Didisheim P: Circulatory Support 1991. The Second International Conference on Circulatory Support for Severe Heart Failure. Infections, prophylaxis and treatment. Ann Thorac Surg 1993;55(1)217–221.
51. Gristina AG, Dobbins JJ, Giammara B, Lewis JC, DeVries WC: Biomaterial-centered sepsis and the total artificial heart: Microbial adhesion vs. tissue integration. JAMA 1988;259(6):870–4.
52. Dobbins JJ, Johnson GS, Kunin CM, DeVries WC: Postmortum microbiological findings of two total artificial heart recipients. JAMA 1988;259(6):865–9.
53. Kunin CM, Dobbins JJ, Melo JC, Levinson MM, Love K, Joyce LD, DeVries WC: Infectious complications in four long-term recipients of the Jarvik-7 artificial heart. JAMA 1988;259(6):860–4.

PREFERRED READING LIST

Ott RA, Gutfinger DE, Gazzaniga AB (ed): Mechanical Cardiac Assist: Cardiac Surgery: State of the Art Reviews. Hanley and Belfus, Inc., Philadelphia, PA 1993;7(2).

Quaal SJ (ed): Cardiac Mechanical Assistance Beyond Balloon Pumping. Mosby, St. Louis, MO 1993.

Bregman D: Mechanical Support of the Failing Heart: Current Problems in Surgery: Year Book Medical Publishers, Inc., Chicago, IL, 1976;XIII(12).

Aufiero TX, Pae WE: Extracorporeal Cardiopulmonary Support for Resuscitation and Invasive Cardiology Outside the Operating Suite. In Gravlee GP, Davis RF, Utley JR (eds): Cardiopulmonary Bypass: Principles and Practice. Williams and Wilkins, Baltimore, MD, 1993:682–692.

Arabia FA, Copeland JG, Larson DF, Smith RG, Cleavinger MR: Circulatory Assist Devices: Applications for Ventricular Recovery or Bridge to Transplant, In Gravlee GP, Davis RF, Utley JR (eds): Cardiopulmonary Bypass: Principles and Practice. Williams and Wilkins, Baltimore, MD, 1993:693–712.

Kesselbrenner M, Sack J, Saporito RA, Bregman D: Intra-aortic Balloon Counterpulsation. In Kay PH (ed): Techniques in Extracorporeal Circulation. Butterworth-Heinemann Ltd, Oxford, UK. Third Edition. 1992:236–267.

Locke T, McGregor C: Ventricular Assist Devices. In Kay PH (ed): Techniques in Extracorporeal Circulation. Butterworth-Heinemann Ltd, Oxford, UK. Third Edition. 1992:268–281.

Bojar RM: Circulatory Assist Devices. In Bojar RM: Adult Cardiac Surgery. Blackwell Scient. Publ., Cambridge, MA, 1992:425–459.

Magovern JA, Pierce WS: Mechanical Circulatory Assistance Before Heart Transplantation, in Baumgartner WA, Reitz BA, Achuff SC (eds): Heart and Heart-Lung Transplantation. W.B. Saunders Company, Philadelphia, PA, 1990:73–85.

ECMO IN THE 90'S

Sherry C. Faulkner, C.C.P.

Arkansas Children's Hospital
Little Rock, Arkansas

The successful use of extracorporeal membrane oxygenation (ECMO) for cardiorespiratory support in a neonate marked the beginning of a new era in the treatment of critically ill patients with respiratory and cardiac dysfunction[1], and started the development of neonatal ECMO centers across the United States and the world. Realizing that the successful growth of neonatal ECMO would require large scale collection of data, Bartlett and Toomasian established the ECMO Registry at the University of Michigan, Ann Arbor, MI and were instrumental in the charter meeting of 65 ECMO centers in September 1989, which led to the creation of the Extracorporeal Life Support Organization (ELSO).

ELSO maintains the ECMO registry and sponsors multicenter studies of new techniques such as veno-venous ECMO support, extracorporeal CO_2 removal, intravascular oxygenation (IVOX), mobile ECMO, and ECMO for cardiac support. This chapter presents an overview of the data provided by ELSO centers over the last four years with major emphasis on cardiac ECMO.

Table 1. ELSO* Neonatal Data.

Neonatal Diagnosis	Survival
Congenital Diaphragmatic Hernia	58%
Meconium Aspiration Syndrome	93%
PPHN/PFC	83%
RDS/HMD	84%
Pneumonia/Sepsis	76%
Air Leak Syndrome	66%
Other	

* Extracorporeal Life Support Organization, ECLS Registry, University of Michigan, Ann Arbor, MI; PPHN/PFC = persistent pulmonary hypertension of neonate, persistent fetal circulation; RDS/HMD = respiratory distress syndrome, hyaline membrane disease

NEONATAL ECMO

Presently the ELSO registry for neonatal ECMO contains data from over 8000 neonates with an overall survival rate greater than 80 percent (table 1).

The inclusion criteria for neonatal ECMO (Table 2) includes gestational age greater than 35 weeks due to the risk of intracranial hemorrhage during heparinization.[2] However, advances in ECMO techniques have lead to studies of ECMO in patients with gestational age less than 34 weeks and birth weight less than 2.0 kg and many centers will now accept neonates with Grade I intracranial hemorrhage as potential ECMO candidates.[3,4] The right heart drainage is accomplished by gravity and requires the elevation of the patient's bed to allow the desired ECMO blood flow of approximately 120 mL/min or 80 to 90 percent of the neonates cardiac output. This high flow results in a narrowed pulse pressure but supports an SaO_2 of 100 percent and systemic venous saturation of 70 to 75 percent.

Table 2. Inclusion Criteria for Neonatal ECMO.

Birth weight > 2.0 kg
Gestational age > 35 weeks
No major bleeding problems
Mechanical ventilation < 10 days
Normal head ultrasound
Reversible pulmonary pathology

Although veno-arterial support predominates, venous-venous ECMO utilizing a double lumen cannula placed in the right internal jugular is more frequently used even for neonates with associated cardiac dysfunction.[5] Currently, there is only one 14 French cannula commercially available in the United States which limits the use of veno-venous extracorporeal life support (ECLS) to patients of the appropriate size.[6] Venous blood is gravity drained through the side holes and the end hold of one lumen while oxygenated blood is returned by the second lumen and directed toward the tricuspid valve through positioning of the side holes. The mixing of oxygenated and deoxygenated blood in the right atrium results in inaccuracies of the venous line saturation as indication of adequate perfusion of the tissue. Veno-venous ECMO requires blood flows initially as high as 150 mL/min and usually result in higher pre-membrane pressure due to the smaller arterial lumen. The patient's arterial pulse pressure will remain wide and the pulse oximetry may read in the low 90%. Originally, it was felt that the patients supported with veno-venous must have good cardiac function. New data suggest that veno-venous can be successfully used on neonates with circulatory compromise. Veno-venous ECMO is advantageous to neonatal patients since the carotid artery is not cannulated, although many ECMO centers will repair the carotid artery following veno-arterial support.[7,8]

Table 3. ELSO* Data.

Population	Survival
Pediatric	
Bacterial pneumonia	47%
Viral pneumonia	50%
Intrapulmonary hemorrhage	62%
Aspiration	58%
Pneumocystis	29%
ARDS	45%
Other	47%
Adult	
Cardiac surgery	42%
Cardiac transplant	40%
Myocarditis	58%
Cardiomyopathy	63%
Other	60%

* Extracorporeal Life Support Organization, ECLS Registry, University of Michigan, Ann Arbor, MI; ARDS = adult respiratory distress syndrome.

PEDIATRIC/ADULT ECMO

Survival of pediatric and adult patients treated with ECMO for respiratory failure does not reach those of the neonate (Table 3). Patient selection is extremely difficult. Most centers still use the original NIH criteria[9] of a transpulmonary shunt greater than 30 percent despite optimal ventilator setting and pharmacological management.

It is generally felt that 2 to 3 days at higher ventilator settings and oxygen requirement is the maximal grace period within which older patients can be placed on ECMO. Use of veno-arterial or veno-venous support depends on the patients cardiac stability. It is not uncommon for veno-venous support to be converted to veno-arterial due to increasing oxygen demand.[10] Surgical approach is varied along with cannulae use. Pediatric and adult ECMO generally are much longer in duration, higher in intensity, and less apt to be successful.[11,12]

CARDIAC ECMO

Cardiac ECMO cases listed in the ELSO Registry total 939 from 1986 to the present with a survival rate of 47 percent (Table 3). No criteria for cardiac ECMO has been established. At Arkansas Children's Hospital we have established protocols for cardiac ECMO.[13,14] These include elimination of residual surgically amendable defects before ECMO in patients failing to wean from cardiopulmonary bypass, and aggressive handling of hemostasis. Administration of platelets before the patient is weaned from conventional cardiopulmonary bypass to ECMO, and rapid infusion of platelets once the patient is on ECMO followed by cryoprecipate greatly assists in stabilizing hemostasis.[15]

Cannulation of the right carotid artery and jugular vein is preferred over mediastinal cannulation to reduce the risk of infection, while the chest incision is left open but covered with an iodinized adhesive. Re-exploration is routinely performed every 36 to 48 hours or more often if needed. During the re-exploration tribiotic or Dakon solution is used for irrigation. Special attention is paid to any signs of bleeding as cardiac tamponade can occur posteriorly despite the open chest incision and what appears to be a dry anterior pericardial sac.

Treatment of left ventricular failure initially requires to totally unload the heart for an extended period of time. Severe left ventricular failure may require a vent placed in the left atrium.[16] Weaning is begun by removal of the left-sided vent followed by slowly decreasing ECMO flow with a concomitantly increase in left ventricular stroke volume. Treatment of hypercontractile right ventricle associated with a reduced stroke volume is achieved by maintaining higher filling volume in the right ventricle through higher central venous pressures.[17] Serial echocardiograms are performed throughout all cardiac supports and assist procedures to determine when the patient is ready for a *trial-off*. The *trial-off* will last at least one hour to assure the patient remains stable off ECMO, an echocardiogram can also be performed at least 20 minutes into the *trial-off*. Following successful *trial-off*, the patient is decannulated. Should the patient later deteriorate or develop problems after a subsequent surgery, there is always a possibility to successfully support a second time with ECMO.

Neonates with cardiac defects that are felt to be correctable as documented by echocardiogram but who are unable to be stabilized medically have been placed on ECMO before cardiac catheterization or surgery.[18] Cardiac surgery can even be performed during ECMO. Depending upon the defect, the patient can be supported with moderate hypothermia and low pump flow or deep hypothermia with circulatory arrest, although most patients with complex defects are transferred to conventional cardiopulmonary bypass for surgical repair while the ECMO cannulae remain in place should ECMO be warranted following repair.

MOBILE ECMO

Mobile ECMO is currently offered by a limited number of centers in the United States.[19-22] Select patients that are too unstable for transport to a regional ECMO center can have the equipment brought to them. There are certainly added risks to not only the patient but also the transport team.

Response time by the ECMO team is of the utmost importance since the patient usually has qualified for ECMO before the referring call is placed. To assure a rapid response, a check list of equipment and task assignments is performed at Arkansas Children's Hospital. The ECMO circuit is primed with crystalloid so that the patient can be placed on support within 30 minutes after reaching the referring hospital. In extreme emergencies, the pump can be primed during flight or ground transport to the referring hospital. All patients are supported with veno-arterial ECMO during transport.

The roller pump utilized at Arkansas Children's Hospital has been modified to allow easy loading into a helicopter or a Lear jet's 36" cargo door. Invertors adapt the aircraft's internal electricity to be compatible with the roller pump. The roller pump does have a 3 to 4 hour battery pack that is used to transport the patient from the ICU to aircraft or van. All accessory equipment such as activated clotting time machine have extended battery life.

ECMO FUTURE

The future of ECMO is boundless. Heparin-bonded circuit for conventional bypass are available in the United States at the current time. While currently not FDA approved, heparin-bonded circuits are being utilized in Europe and other parts of the world for ECMO and are under investigation in the United States. Such circuits would open the door for support of premature infants and trauma patients. The ECMO pumps continue to evolve. While most centers rely on a roller pump with servo-regulation by a bladder box plunger technique, servo-regulation by monitoring pressure gives the additional information of the volume status and return to the pump. This is extremely important in the treatment of the cardiac ECMO patient. Future pump developments include the AREC veno-venous pump utilized in Europe, where blood flow is generated by an alternating clamp on the non-occlusive pump.[23] Other future developments include hollow-fiber oxygenators and Intravascular Oxygenation (IVOX, CardioPulmonics, Salt Lake City, UT). The IVOX has shown limited ability to oxygenate blood, yet is very promising in the removal of CO_2.[24] Multi-center trials are in progress throughout the world at this time. The use of inhaled nitric oxide for neonates and cardiac patients is gaining popularity and may actually eliminate the need for ECMO in select patients.[25] Liquid ventilation with perfluorocarbon solutions is being used in conjunction with ECMO in an animal model by Hirschl and colleagues.[26] Intratracheal pulmonary ventilation (ITPV) is currently being used by a few centers to either support patients before qualifying for ECMO or to assist with weaning from ECMO. Research regarding ITPV continues under the guidance of Theordor Kolobow.[27]

While Bartlett's first successful neonatal ECMO led to rapid advancements in ECMO over a short period of time, the future of ECMO is equally as bright.

REFERENCES

1. Extracorporeal life support. Arensman RM, Cornish JD (eds). Blackwell Scientific Publications, 1993:32–33.
2. Chapman RA, Toomasian JM, Bartlett RH: Extracorporeal Membrane Oxygenation, Technical Manual, 7th Edition, University of Michigan Medical Center, 1991.
3. Marsh TD, Visser V, Duncan S, Cook L: Risk of intraventricular hemorrhage in 33–34 week ECMO patients. 7th Annual Children's National Medical Center ECMO Symposium. February 1991:32 (Abstract).
4. Hirschl RB, Schumacher R, Snedecor S, Bartlett RH: The efficacy of ECLS in premature and low birth weight newborns. 8th Annual Children's National Medical Center ECMO Symposium. February 1992:61 (Abstract).
5. Cornish JD, Heiss KF, Clark RH, Rickett RP, Parker P, Boecler B, Kisser K, Streper M: Preferential use of venovenous ECMO for neonates with significant circulatory compromise. 8th Annual Children's National Medical Center ECMO symposium. February 1992:87 (Abstract).

6. Perreault T, Johnston A, Morneault L, Mullahoo K, Adolph V: Use of a twelve French double lumen catheter in newborns supported with extracorporeal membrane oxygenation (ECMO). 5th Annual Extracorporeal Life Support Organization. October 1993:22 (Abstract).
7. Taylor BJ, Seibert JJ, Van Devanter SH, Harrell JE, Fasules JW: Evaluation of the reconstructed carotid artery following extracorporeal membrane oxygenation. Pediat 1992;90:568–572.
8. Whittlesey GC, Becker C, Meyer SL, Klein MD: MRI evaluation following cervical vessel ligation. 5th Annual Extracorporeal Life Support Organization. October 1993:49 (Abstract).
9. Zapol WM, Snider MT, Hill DJ, et al: Extracorporeal membrane oxygenation in severe acute respiratory failure: A randomized prospective study. JAMA 1979;242:2193–6.
10. Anderson HL, Attori RJ, Custer JR, Chapman RA, Bartlett RH: Extracorporeal membrane oxygenation for pediatric cardiopulmonary failure. J Thorac Cardiovasc Surg 1990;99:1011–21.
11. Moler F, Palmisano J, Custer J, Akingbola O, Bartlett R: ECLS for severe pediatric respiratory failure: An updated experience 1991–1993. 5th Annual Extracorporeal Life Support Organization. October 1993:11 (Abstract).
12. Karlson KH, Pickert CB, Schexnayder SM, Heulitt MJ: Flexible fiberoptic bronchoscopy in children on ECMO. Pediatric Pulmonology. (In Press)
13. Faulkner SC, Chipman CW, Moss MM, Frazier EA, Fasules JW, Harrell JE, Ziomek S, VanDevanter SH: Techniques utilized for extracorporeal membrane oxygenation (ECMO) support of postoperative pediatric cardiac patients. Proceedings of Am Acad of Cardiovasc Perf 1992;13:32–35.
14. Ziomek S, Harrell JE, Fasules JW, Faulkner S, Chipman C, Moss MM, Frazier EA, VanDevanter SH: Cardiopulmonary failure following congenital heart surgery: results of treatment with extracorporeal membrane oxygenation. Ann Thorac Surg (In Press)
15. Faulkner SC, Baker LL, Kletzel M, Fasules JW, Taylor BJ: Effects on platelet count and function utilizing two different methods of platelet transfusion during extracorporeal membrane oxygenation (ECMO) support. 3rd Extracorporeal Life Support Organization. September 1991:33 (Abstract).
16. Zwischenberger JB, Cox CS: ECMO in the management of cardiac failure. ASAIO 1992:751–753.
17. Frazier EA, Moss MM, Faulkner SC, VanDevanter SH: Postoperative extracorporeal membrane oxygenation for decreased right ventricular stroke volume in congenital heart patients. 4th Extracorporeal Life Support Organization. October 1992:33 (Abstract).
18. Faulkner SC, Chipman CW, Moss MM, Frazier EA, Bushman GA, Fasules JW, Love JC, Harrell JE, VanDevanter SH: Extracorporeal life support of neonates with congenital cardiac defects: techniques used during cardiac catheterization and surgery. JECT (In Press).
19. Cornish JD, Gerstmann DR, Begnaudd MJ, Null DM, Ackerman NB: Inflight use of extracorporeal membrane oxygenation for severe neonatal respiratory failure. Perfusion 1986;1:281–287.
20. Long WB, Hill J, Bruhn PS, Irwin LM, Everson S, Pearson UJ, Matar AF: Helicopter transportation of a critically ill patient on a portable cardiopulmonary bypass system. 2nd Extracorporeal Life Support Organization. November 1990:38 (Abstract).
21. Shapiro MB, Anderson H, MacDonald GA, Remenapp RE, Chapman RA, Bartlett RH: Mobile extracorporeal life support (ECLS) for critically unstable patients. 4th Extracorporeal Life Support Organization. October 1992:73 (Abstract).
22. Faulkner SC, Taylor BJ, Chipman CW, Baker LL, Fasules JW, VanDevanter SH, Harrell JE: Mobile extracorporeal membrane oxygenation. Ann Thorac Surg 1993;55:1244–1246.
23. Chevalier JY, Renolleau S, Couprie C, Durandy Y, Mathe JC, Costil J: The use of AREC/extracorporeal: CO_2 removal an alternative to neonatal veno-arterial ECMO. 4th Extracorporeal Life Support Organization. October 1992:48 (Abstract).
24. Schaap RN, Gaykowski R, Mortensen JD: Results to date of the clinical trials of the intravenacaval oxygenator (IVOX). 3rd Annual Extracorporeal Life Support Organization. September 1991:55.

25. Finer NN, Etches PC, Kamstra B, Tierney AJ, Peliowski A, Ryan CA: Inhaled nitric oxide in infants referred for ECMO: dose response. 3rd Annual Extracorporeal Life Support Organization. September 1991:14.
26. Hirschl RB, Tooley R, Parent A, Johnson K, Bartlett RH: Partial liquid ventilation improves gas exchange in the setting of respiratory failure during extracorporeal life support (ECLS). 5th Annual Extracorporeal Life Support Organization. October 1993:8.
27. Aprigliano M, Kolobow T, Rossi N, Tsuno K: Intratracheal pulmonary ventilation (ITPV), and continuous positive pressure ventilation (CPPV) in a sheep model of acute respiratory failure. A controlled, randomized study. 5th Annual Extracorporeal Life Support Organization. October 1993:12.

RADIOFREQUENCY ABLATION OF VENTRICULAR TACHYCARDIA

Joan M. Craney, R.N., M.S.N.

Boston College School of Nursing
Boston, MA

Radiofrequency ablation (RFA) of ventricular tachycardia (VT) is a new treatment for hemodynamically destablizing sustained VT. Although not considered a treatment for all types of VT, RFA does have its place next to antiarrhythmic medication, implantable cardioverter defibrillator, and cardiothoracic surgery for certain persistent types of VT.[1]

PATIENT POPULATION AT RISK

Generally, patients with a history of heart disease are prone to VT because of diffuse areas of endocardial injury which can serve as substrate for VT. Eighty percent of patients have a history of coronary artery disease, and/or prior myocardial infarction.[2] Another 15 percent have a history of cardiomyopathy or congestive heart failure. The remaining 5 percent present with no cardiac pathology. Most patients have a decreased ejection fraction, have smoked cigarettes in the past or are presently smoking, have an ECG showing either premature ventricular contractions, sustained or nonsustained VT with multiple morphologies, and may have a ventricular aneurysm. The majority of patients present with multiple complaints of syncope or palpitations, and prior cardiac arrest.[3,4]

According to the 1990 American Heart Association statistics, 500,000 people die each year from sudden cardiac death due to VT or ventricular fibrillation (VF). Those who survive may have recurrences of VT/VF, display multiple cardiac morphologies, and may be severely hemodynamically compromised. If left untreated, patients with sustained VT have a 40 percent mortality rate at one year. These patients are generally noted to have a left ventricular aneurysm or scar.[5]

A second group of patients who experience VT are those with normal hearts but with either mitral valve prolapse, right ventricular dysplasia, hypertrophy, or idiopathic congenital heart disease such as Ebstein's anomaly and Tetralogy of Fallot. These patients tend to be younger in age, and because of normal heart function, they tolerate the fast heart rates of VT and are more frequently amenable to RFA then patients with cardiac disease.

MECHANISMS OF VENTRICULAR TACHYCARDIA

Re-entry is the most common cause of VT. It occurs when an impulse, produced by the normal conduction system, returns to restimulate myocardial tissue and continues to restimulate previously excited tissues. Three criteria must be present for the re-entry phenomenon to exist.[6]
1. unidirectional block in the electrical circuit of the heart
2. an area of slowed conduction or ischemia
3. the tissue at the site of the block can accept the impulse and re-excite the myocardial tissue, causing conduction to occur as a circular or *circus* movement.

Heart rates that become excessively fast, can deteriorate into VF. *Enhanced automaticity* is a repeated generation of an impulse by one or more ectopic foci outside the normal sequence of conduction. Enhanced activity can be produced by electrolyte abnormalities, or enhanced sympathetic nervous system activity.[6]

CONVENTIONAL TREATMENT MODALITIES

Antiarrhythmic medication is typically the first line of treatment for VT/VF. Class 1A agents such as, procainamide, quinidine, and mexiletine are prescribed first and if ineffective, a class 1C agent, such as propafenone, or class III agents such as amiodarone and sotalol are recommended. The efficacy rate for medication in the treatment of VT/VF is reported to be 40 percent. Of those for whom the medication is effective, many report side effects such as diarrhea, nausea, and vomiting.

Implantable cardioverter defibrillator (ICD) are becoming more common for the treatment of VT/VF. Twenty-five thousand devices have been implanted since 1980. Once implanted, the ICD can reduce the mortality to less than 3 percent at one year. A majority of these patients may require medication in addition to their ICD. A small portion of these patients have frequent episodes of VT which are not controlled by medication. In this case, they utilize their ICD often, are in jeopardy of depleting the battery life, thus necessitating early replacement.

A third method of treatment is cardiothoracic surgery. Patients who would benefit from this procedure are patients with VT/VF which is resistant to drug therapy, patients who displayed a toxicity or allergy to antiarrhythmic medication, or patients who have compelling reason for other surgery such as triple vessel disease necessitating coronary artery bypass grafting (CABG).[5] The goal of cardiothoracic surgery is the removal of the pathophysiological basis for the arrhythmia, localization and ablation of the substrate, and the exclusion, isolation or confinement of the arrhythmogenic zone.[7]

Cardiothoracic procedures with potential beneficial effect for the treatment of VT/VF are CABG, subendocardial resection (SER), cryoablation and aneurysmectomy.

CABG itself has an approximately 56 percent success rate in treating VT.[7] SER, developed in 1979 to treat VT refractory to drug therapy, depends on accurate intraoperative endocardial mapping to localize the arrhythmogenic area that produces VT. The procedure consists of resection of the region of endocardial fibrosis. SER is the most widely used procedure for ischemic VT, but it is not effective with multiple morphologic VT's that require time to map and resect.[7-9] SER is also not initiated for patients with poor left ventricular function because these patients are at high surgical risk.[9] In these cases, non-thoracotomy ICD placement or an RFA procedure are generally recommended.[10] Cryoablation is primarily an adjunctive therapy to be used with SER. This technique is versatile, precise, it can be rapidly applied and it preserves tissue collagen and ventricular wall integrity.[11] Aneurysmectomy requires mapping of the edge of the aneurysm and excision of the area of arrhythmogenic foci.[8]

RADIOFREQUENCY ABLATION

RFA may be used for patients who are:
1) too ill for surgery such as SER because of a low ejection fraction (less than 20 percent) or a high surgical risk,[3] 2) those with multiple morphologies, especially slow VT that can be mapped in the electrophysiology laboratory without hemodynamic compromise,[3] and 3) for those with an already implanted ICD but have frequent episodes of tachycardia which often require pace termination or defibrillation.[3]

RFA PROCEDURE

RFA involves the delivery of radiofrequency energy, through a steerable pacing catheter to the targeted tissue site. High frequency current is passed between the distal electrode of the catheter and a large diameter grounding pad, generally placed at the level of the right scapula. With energy application, the temperature of the contact tissue rises, water is driven out, and coagulation necrosis results. Repeated applications of radiofrequency energy are often necessary until the morphologic VT disappears during RFA, VT is not reproducible, and/or a sharp impedance rise occurs indicating coagulum formation on the ablating electrode.

The exact amount of tissue injury depends on the energy delivered (20 to 30 watts or higher), the duration of delivery (60 sec), and the impedance (N=100 ohms). The delivered energy and its duration can be controlled to achieve the desired effect on the tissue. This results in small and controllable lesions since the system delivers localized heat rather than large poorly localized burns.

ADVANTAGES OF RFA

RFA is performed without general anesthesia. This represents a major advantage since neuromuscular fibers are not stimulated, pain receptors are not stimulated by the radiofrequency energy. The incidence of proarrhythmia (less than 0.2 percent) and the risk of perforation of myocardium is low (less than 2 percent), as little damage is done to the surrounding tissue. The catheter tip impedance is closely monitored and the delivery of energy is terminated for any sudden rise. In this case, the catheter is usually removed, cleaned and reinserted to continue the procedure. The procedure takes place in the electrophysiology (EPS) laboratory where pre-gelled external defibrillation pads are placed in the anterior-posterior position. Both inguinal, and the right internal jugular areas are prepared in a sterile fashion. The procedure is performed under conscious sedation (midazolam hydrochloride) and pain control (Meperidine). Some centers intubate the patient in order to be able to obtain a deeper level of sedation.

Cardiac catheterization is performed under a local anesthetic. Pacing catheters are positioned in the right ventricle, right atrium, or AV node. Another catheter is positioned at the site to be ablated and an attempt is made to initiate VT with ventricular burst pacing. In most instances, this is easily accomplished since patients experience numerous spontaneous VT episodes and often remain in a hemodynamically stable VT throughout the procedure.

IDENTIFICATION AND DETECTION OF VT FOCI

In order to identify the origin of the VT, the heart is paced at different sites until a nearly identical ECG is produced that matches the clinical VT. The ablating catheter's electrogram should show the earliest activation to be greater than 30 msec before the surface QRS. In addition, there should be a discreet potential present during diastole while in VT and a so-called *concealed entrainment* which represents the tachycardia at 30 to 100 msec greater than the rate of tachycardia.[2-4,12]

Once the site is localized, the distal electrode of the ablating catheter is connected to the radiofrequency generator. Radiofrequency energy is then applied in an attempt to obliterate the VT. Each application can last 10 to 60 seconds at 15 to 30 watts, with a normal measured impedance of approximately 100 ohms.

COMPLICATIONS

Despite the relative safety of ablation with radiowaves, complications may occur. The procedure is associated with a slight increase in creatinine phosphokinase (CPK) as intentional myocardial necrosis occurs. This should not be a cause for concern. Other complications include cardiac tamponade (less than 1 percent), deep vein thrombosis (less than 1 percent), VT at a faster rate, chest discomfort, trauma to vessels (less than 1 percent require surgical intervention), transient ischemic attack and/or stroke (less than 0.5 percent), and hematoma at introducer site (common, usually without sequelae)[13]

NURSING CARE DURING RFA PROCEDURE

During RFA procedure, nursing care focuses on prevention of complications and safety measures such as: 1) *Reduction of anxiety*, especially when episodes of tachycardia occur. For some patients, episodes of tachycardia are frightening and signify a loss of control. Reassurance must be given with each episode. 2) *Prevention of thrombosis*. Heparin is administered to prevent thrombosis formation and embolization. High-range activated clotting times are monitored every hour to maintain clotting times above 300 sec. 3) *Patient safety while under sedation*. All patients receiving sedation require careful monitoring of blood pressure, heart rate, respiratory rate, and arterial oxygen saturation throughout the procedure. Nasal oxygen is administered, as needed to maintain adequate SaO_2 greater than 95 percent, especially during tachycardia events, or during cardiac pacing.[13]

POST-ABLATION NURSING CARE

After the ablation, all venous and arterial pacing catheters are removed. If cardiac tamponade is suspected, an echocardiogram is performed to document the presence of any pericardial fluid that may have accumulated as a result of perforation. Vital signs, along with peripheral extremity pulse checks, and groin checks for hematomas, are performed routinely. Strict bedrest is maintained until the next morning. The patient's heart rhythm is monitored in the event VT should recur. Anti-arrhythmic medication is resumed if necessary for untreated VT morphologies. Within a few days, patients return to the EPS laboratory for a repeat study. Induction of the VT is attempted via pacing catheters positioned in the right ventricle. Most patients are monitored in the hospital for 5 to 10 days before discharge.

FOLLOW-UP

Long-term follow-up consists of arrhythmia clinic visits every 2 to 3 months. Most patients may also have an ICD which should be assessed during the same visit.

LIMITATIONS OF RFA IN VT

Patients eligible for RFA represent only 10 percent of the population presenting with VT.[3] RFA is not always successful in eliminating all arrhythmogenic foci for VT. Generally, one or two of the morphologies can be eliminated and, in most cases, adjunctive therapy such as an ICD or antiarrhythmic medication is necessary.[3] Despite these limitations, RFA of VT should be considered for treatment of patients with hemodynamically destablizing sustained VT, who are not candidates for surgery, whose VT is resistant to medication, and who are receiving multiple appropriate ICD shocks for VT.

FUTURE CONSIDERATIONS

Improvements in the RFA procedure can be made through advanced designs in steerable ablating catheters. Better control and manipulation of the catheter tip can facilitate the RFA procedure and aid in the localization of areas of arrhythmogenic foci. Research and development in radiofrequency generator's energy delivery and temperature control will allow more precise and less traumatic lesions. RFA is an exciting new therapy, however, caution is warranted to maximize patient safety and assess long-term complications.

REFERENCES

1. Stevens LL, Redd RM, Buckingham TA: Emergency catheter ablation of refractory ventricular tachycardia. CCN 1989;9(5):36–40.
2. Morady F: Catheter ablation of ventricular tachycardia. In Josephson ME and Wellens HJJ (Eds.) Tachycardias: Mechanisms and Management. The Futura Publishing Co., Inc., Mount Kisko, NY, 1993:537–556.
3. Morady F, Harvey M, Kalbfleisch SJ, El-Atassis R, Calkins H, Langberg J: Radiofrequency catheter ablation of ventricular tachycardia in patients with coronary artery disease. Circulation 1993;87(2):363–372.
4. Gursoy S, Chiladakis I, Kuck KH: First lessons from radiofrequency catheter ablation in patients with ventricular tachycardia. PACE 1993;16:687–691.
5. Cox JL: Surgical management of cardiac arrhythmias. In McGoon D (Eds.) Cardiovascular Clinics: Cardiac Surgery. F.A. Davis, Co., Philadelphia, PA, 1987:770–821.
6. Bigger JT: Ventricular arrhythmias: classification and general principles of therapy. In Horowitz LN (Eds.), Current Management of Arrhythmias. B.C. Decker, Inc., Philadelphia, PA, 1991:130–137.
7. Boineau JP, Cox JL: Rationale for a direct surgical approach to control arrhythmias. Am J Cardiol 1982;49:381–396.
8. Josephson ME, Harken AH, Horowitz LN: Endocardial excision: a new surgical technique for the treatment of recurrent ventricular tachycardia. Circulation 1979;60(7):1430–1439.
9. Miller JM, Kienzle MD, Harken AH, Josephson ME: Subendocardial resection for ventricular tachycardias: predictors of surgical success. Circulation 1984;70(4):624–631.
10. Trappe HJ, Klein H, Wenzlaff P, Frank G, Siclari F, Gotte A, Lichtlen PR: Ventricular tachycardia surgery in 1992: did the automatic defibrillator change this approach? PACE 1993;16:242–246.
11. Ferguson TB, Cox JL: Antiarrhythmic surgery: Ventricular arrhythmias. In Horowitz LN (Eds.), Current Management of Arrhythmias. B.C. Decker, Inc., Philadelphia, PA, 1991:382–391.
12. Page RL, Shenasa H, Evans JJ, Sorrentino RA, Wharton JM, Prystowsky EN: Radiofrequency catheter ablation of idiopathic recurrent ventricular tachycardia with right bundle branch block, left axis morphology. PACE 1993;16:327–336.
13. Craney JM: Radiofrequency catheter ablation of supraventricular tachycardia: Clinical considerations and nursing care. J Cardiovasc Nursing 1993;7(3):26–39.

UPDATE IN INTERNAL CARDIOVERTER DEFIBRILLATORS

Julia Ann Purcell, R.N., M.N., C.C.R.N.

Emory University Hospital
Atlanta, Georgia

This chapter will describe some of the major technological advances in the field of internal cardioverter defibrillator (ICD) therapy. In 1993, the Food and Drug Administration (FDA) approved the release of two transvenous leads, allowing the majority of ICD patients less intrusive surgery and a reduced length of hospital stay and shortened recovery time. (see appendix A). In addition, the third generation pulse generators were released, extending the advantage of tiered therapies to a broader patient population. These devices can not only defibrillate and cardiovert, but also have the capability of back-up ventricular demand pacing, anti-tachycardia pacing (ATP) (burst or rapid overdrive pacing) and sophisticated programming options for ECG sensing and delivery of shocks and/or pacing stimuli (Table 1).

Appropriately ATP often allows a painless conversion of slower types of monomorphic ventricular tachyarrhythmia. Moreover, back-up ventricular pacing can prevent episodes of tachyarrhythmia occurring in association with bradyarrhythmia. A few ICD patients require a separate permanent pacemaker when battery depletion is anticipated by extensive use since usual pacing requires the same pulse/width and pulse/amplitude settings as for burst pacing conversion of ventricular tachyarrhythmia. Amongst other advantages, newer ICD pulse generators are expected to have greater sophistication in pacing-mode options, as well as independent energy settings for back-up and ATP pacing.

Improvements in the delivery of electrical therapy have also been made as biphasic shock waveforms are replacing monophasic shock waveforms of earlier generation ICD's. However most patients continue to report significant discomfort with any form of shock therapy for ventricular fibrillation, polymorphic ventricular tachycardia (multiple QRS shapes), rapid rate monomorphic ventricular tachycardia less than 170/minute, or episodes of tachyarrhythmia unresponsive to anti-tachycardia pacing.

Until it is possible to convert such rhythms with significantly lower energy, the decision to place an ICD implies a responsibility to assist the

Table 1. Reference Chart for Internal Cardioverter Defibrillators

Model/Weight	# Shocks/episode	On/Off Mechanism	Follow-up Reforming Capacitors	Life Expectancy	Programming	Brady-Pacing	Anti-tachycardia Pacing	Interrogation
CPI (St. Paul, MN)								
Ventak* P-2 1625 (233 g)	300/can (5/episode)	Programmer preferred for usual "on/off" adjustments. Magnet will convert from "on" to "off" in an emergency (if applied to R corner of pulse generator for 30 sec.)	Programmer used to stimulate occurrence of one shock delivered to pulse generator (to reform capacitors) every 2 months from implant to end of life.	5.8 years	Extensive options VT/VF Zones, rates duration, polarity, waveform, VVI and post-shock pacing.	Brady, VVI post-shock pacing.	None	2035 programmer and software module.
Ventak 1520 (240 g)	100/can (4/episode)	Magnet over R-side pulse generator for 30 sec will convert from "on" to "off" or vice versa	5 second magnet application over R corner pulse generator causes one shock build-up with discharge required every 2 months for 1st year, then every month until replacement	2–3 years	None	None	None	Using Aid-check during magnet tests, can determine # shocks given to patient (must keep records of # chocks used with magnet tests)
Ventak 1550 (235 g)	300/can (5/episode)	Programmer preferred for usual "on/off" adjustments. Magnet will convert pulse generator to "off" or "on" in an emergency (if applied to R corner of pulse generator for 30 sec.)	Programmer used to reform capacitors every 2 months from implant to end of life (causes one shock to be delivered to can.)	5.8 years	Limited programmability, i.e., rate cutoff, 1st shock joules, etc.	None	None	Using programmer, can determine both # of shocks delivered to patient AND # of magnet tests/current settings (rate cutoff, joules for each shock, etc.)
Ventak P 1600 (235 g)	300/can (5/episode)	Programmer preferred for usual "on/off" adjustments. Magnet will convert from "on" to "off" in an emergency (if applied to R corner of pulse generator for 30 sec.)	Programmer used to stimulate occurrence of one shock delivered to pulse generator (to reform capacitors) every 2 months from implant to end of life.	5.8 years	Programmability for tach. rate cut-off, 2.5 to 10 sec delay in charging from onset of tach, & lower joules	None	None	Same as model 1550

Update in Internal Cardioverter Defibrillators

Manufacturer/Device	Therapy	Shocks/Capacity	Capacitor Reformation	Battery Life	Programming	Bradycardia Pacing	Antitachycardia Pacing	Additional Features
Ventritex (Sunnyvale, CA) Cadence V-100	Tiered therapy	100-300/can	Capacitors are reformed/charged on a programmable schedule.	Programmer used to activate or deactivate device. (Magnet will TEMPORARILY inhibit shocks and antitachycardia pacing when placed over the lower middle of pulse generator.) Magnet does not effect brady pacing.	48-60 months depending on usage	Extensive programming options (#/length of burst pacing shocks, rates, joules, etc.)	Yes	Yes	Ventritex Programmer (in EP Lab). Extensive diagnostic and event recorder with stored electrograms. Non invasive program stimulation.
Telectronics (Denver, CO) Guardian ATP* 4210 (269 g)	530/can (warranted for 250) (Can be set for 4-7 shocks per episode)	Device automatically reforms capacitors every 60 days. (MD follow-up needed during clinical investigation to interrogate device and determine usage.	Programmer used to activate or deactivate device. (Magnet will TEMPORARILY inhibit shocks and antitachycardia pacing when placed over the lower middle of pulse generator.)	Approximately 5 years, depending on usage	Extensive programming options (#/length of burst pacing shocks, rates, joules, etc.)	Yes	Yes (Burst) (Can be programmed to only burst pace and not shock for slower Vtach)	Using programmer, can see past usage (shocks/burst pacing), etc. as well as R-R intervals requiring intervention and follow-up.
Medtronics, Inc. (Minneapolis, MN) PCD (Pacemaker Cardioverter-Defibrillator	350/can 1-4/episode as programmed	Capacitors must be reformed every 3 months by programmer on MD visit.	Programmer used to activate or deactivate device. (Magnet will TEMPORARILY inhibit shocks and antitachycardia pacing when placed over the lower middle of pulse generator.)	Approximately 5 years, depending on usage	Extensive programming options (#/length of burst pacing shocks, rates, joules, etc.)	Yes	Yes (Ramp/decremental and Burst options)	

*Clinical investigation in process in USA

patient in making a long-term emotional adjustment. It seems of utmost importance to provide the referring physician and the office staff with information related to the device, how the ICD can be temporarily turned off if needed, and electrophysiology study-guided recommendations for drug therapy in case there is recurrent repetitive dysrhythmia (appendix B). Moreover, an active patient/family follow-up program is recommended (appendix C). Should a patient require emergency intervention in a site away from his/her home physician, 24-hour call to an electrophysiologist who is familiar with the specific details related to the ICD implant and immediate access to the implant records is essential.

Considering the reduced length of hospital stay, creative ways should be found to help the patient and family understand the characteristics as well as limitations of the implanted ICD during weekly telephone or office visit follow-up during the first 6 to 8 weeks post-implant. The emotional impact of having a complex electrical device within the body is often not evident until several weeks after implant. In some cases, it does not manifest until the reality of the surprise of a first shock(s). When the patient and family confronts this first experience, they need considerable emotional support to process their feelings of surviving a *near death experience*. Although health care personnel are elated on the ICD's success over sudden death, many patients are not totally reassured until they have adequately processed their feelings and have become knowledgeable about the episode. It is essential to let the patient (and the significant other) express details related to the time of the shock and any potential influence of changes in daily activities or medication timing. If a series of shocks occur, one can anticipate considerable psychological trauma. Although ICD support groups are of some value, meticulous medical follow-up is needed to minimize the number of episodes with appropriate drug therapy and tailoring the ICD programming options to the type of dysrhythmia. Research continues in an effort to document the impact of ICD implantation on the quality of life for these individuals as well as defining successful coping aids for the patient and family. Although the length of hospital stay has been reduced, the *tunneling* procedure to connect the transvenous lead to the pulse generator often is associated with discomfort for at least several months, perhaps longer as in the case of a subcutaneous patch. Appropriate medication for this should be offered along with further exploration to minimize the trauma associated with this technique.

Appendix A

ICD INSERTION (EP Lab or OR)

PURPOSE: To prepare patient for insertion of an automatic implantable cardioverter defibrillator (ICD).

PROCEDURE: Implement following pre-ICD standing orders:

1. Draw (or have drawn) blood for lab studies: PLT, CBC, SMA7, PT, and PTT. In addition, a chest x-ray is needed unless one has been done in last 30 days.
2. NPO after Mn except for Meds. ordered by M.D.
3. Start #18 gauge angiocath (or #20 if needed) and cap with a heparin lock in dominant upper extremity.
4. Clip hair and scrub with hibiclens X1 to following: pubic symphysis to neck, anterior right axillary line to left posterior axillary line.
5. Complete pre-operative checklist.
6. Informed consent (signed, witnessed and on chart) by M.D.

DESCRIPTION OF PROCEDURE:

After skin preparation, ECG electrodes and defibrillation gel-pads are placed on the patient. (The EP nurse will refer to these as EKG pads, warning the patient that they feel "cold" for the first couple of seconds). General anesthesia is given (anesthesia personnel) with intubation so testing of the device (induction of tachyarrhythmia/ventricular fibrillation and shocks with the device) can occur without the patient being aware. There are two incisions: the 2-3 inch one near the right subclavian vein (upper chest) and the 3-4 inch incision in the left lower quadrant for the pulse generator. Afterwards, the patient goes to PACU for recovery from the anesthesia until ready to return to their room. An ICU stay is NOT usually required.

PATIENT PREPARATION:

1. Give patient and family copy of appropriate booklets: "Off the Beat", and/or manufacturer's ICD booklet.
2. Complete teaching and document on patient family teaching record.
3. Have family wait in patient room.

POST-PROCEDURE for ICD INSERTION: (Implement pre-printed post-ICD standing orders placed on patient's chart during procedure)

1. Admit to _____
2. ICD is [active or inactive] (circle one) with a rate cutoff of ___beats/minute. The device [will or will not] (circle one) attempt to overdrive pace tachycardia. Back-up brady pacing rate _____ (if applicable).
3. Continuous ECG monitoring with HR alarms for < ___beats/minute or > ___beats per minute.
4. Vital signs q 30 x 4 (or as ordered by M.D.), then per routine. Monitor quality of radial pulse on arm nearest ICD incision. Oral temperature at 8 pm for 48 hours. Inspect incisions for swelling or bleeding with each VS and every 4 hours for 24 hours. Record observations on VS flow sheet.
5. Activity: Bedrest x 6 hours then up ad lib. Check BP lying, sitting, and standing with first ambulation. Patient to avoid lifting arm above shoulder level for 10 days.
6. Upright portable chest x-ray on arrival: "R/O pneumothorax."
7. May place Foley catheter prn for inability to void. Discontinue when patient is ambulatory.
8. IV fluids: Give _____ liters of NS @ 150 cc/hr, then convert IV to Heparin lock.
9. Diet: Progress from clear liquids to previously ordered diet as tolerated.
10. Medications: Resume pre-procedure medications.
    Ciprofloxacin (Cipro) 500 mg PO b.i.d. x 10 doses.
    Nalbuphine (Nubain) 1-2 mg IV q 1 min up to a maximum of 10 mg q 3 hours prn pain.
    Metoclopramide (Reglan) 10 mg IV q 4 hours prn nausea.
    Percocet 1-2 tablets PO q 4 hours prn pain.
11. Notify EP fellow _____ (Pic   ) of (1) bleeding/hematoma, (2) hypotension or narrow pulse pressure, dizziness or weakness, (3) discomfort unrelieved by Percocet, (4) new onset shortness of breath or cyanosis, (5) new onset arrhythmias or any evidence of ICD shocks or rapid pacing, or (6) temperature > 100 degrees (oral).
12. Set-up follow-up appointments. Electrophysiology device testing planned for_____.

Appendix B

_____(date)

Name
Street Address
City, State & Zip Code

To whom it may concern:

[Mr., Mrs., Ms.,]_____, had an internal cardioverter defibrillator implanted on _____(date) at _____ Hospital. The device is made by [Cardiac Pacemaker, Inc. (CPI) [P2 or _____], model _____ or Ventritex Cadence®] and has been programmed to:

    ___ overdrive pace if the heart rate exceeds ___/minute
    ___ deliver one or more shocks [if the heart rate >___/minute] ___ [& rapid pacing is ineffective].
    ___ back-up pace if the heart rate < ___/minute.

A [transvenous or thoracotomy] surgical approach was used to insert the leads/pulse generator. (See ID card for details of lead placement).

The internal defibrillator is _expected_ to terminate any episodes of ventricular tachycardia or ventricular fibrillation. However, if the patient becomes pulseless, treat it like anyone else in that situation. Start CPR immediately and use external defibrillation as soon as any chest muscular contractions cease (from shocks of the ICD). Any shocks from the internal defibrillator occur at the outset of a new rhythm and after providing the designated number of shocks, it will remain "on standby" until there is a change in the rhythm.

If external defibrillation does not revert the rhythm, move the paddles to a new position around the heart. (Anterior-posterior defibrillation may allow the most direct angle in these situations).

If supraventricular tachycardias occur with a fast enough ventricular rate, the ICD will make its usual effort, but it is unlikely the voltage will be enough to convert the patient to sinus rhythm. A large magnet (such as the ones used to check a pacemaker) can be placed over the pulse generator to [temporarily inhibit overdrive pacing or shocks (Medtronic, Telectronics, Ventritex devices)] or [turn off the ICD once in place for 30 seconds (CPI devices)].

We have advised the patient to avoid strong magnetic fields such as:

    -large magnets used in junk yards to move cars or the ones used to move hot steel in a smelting furnace.
    -high voltage power transformers and transmission lines,
    -radio transmitters, walkie-talkie or radio control units for remote toys held within 6" of the pulse generator of the ICD,
    -arc welding.

If properly maintained, usual household appliances and garden/lawn equipment _will not_ interfere with the function of the defibrillator.

We will arrange for follow-up visits to interrogate the device for past operation and to evaluate the battery. At times, testing in the Electrophysiology Laboratory may also be required.

                                Sincerely,

                                M.D.

Appendix C

Discharge Instructions for a Transvenous Internal
Cardioverter Defibrillator (ICD)

Self Care:

You may resume showering 5 days after your ICD surgery (unless there are signs of infection). Although you should allow several weeks for full recovery for ICD surgery, you should expect to return to most of your usual activities. An ICD is like having "extra insurance." You may not ever need it, but if you do, it works right away to try and get your heart back in normal rhythm. Taking your medications exactly as prescribed is the best way to prevent any changes in your heart rhythm. Please do not stop or change the dosage of any of your drugs!

Activities/Limitations/Exercise/Sexual Activity:

It may take 2-3 months for the twinges under your arm to resolve after ICD surgery, particularly if there is a patch under the skin. Most patients resume usual exercise a few weeks after surgery but you are the best judge of how quickly you can go back to all of your activities. We suggest the following:

-Wait about a week before resuming sexual intercourse.
-Gently resume normal usage of the arm nearest the chest incision but during the first 10 days, limit any lifting to less than 10 lbs. and do not raise it above your shoulder. This gives the lead in the heart time to settle in a secure place. After that, be sure to gently exercise the shoulder until you have full range of motion.

If your physician agrees that you may drive, wait about ten days. Some states advise the physician that driving is not permitted in the first year after a fainting spell due to abnormal heart rhythm. Your physician will make a recommendation for you based on the severity of symptoms caused during your abnormal rhythm and the last time an episode occurred. The recommendation would be the same whether you have an ICD or not.

We will test your ICD before discharge from the hospital to be sure it works as expected. Some ICD's can send out fast, painless pacing signals to try and change an abnormal heart rhythm back to normal. However, the shock of an ICD will probably be something you notice (unless the abnormal rhythm causes you to pass out). Some people compare an ICD shock to getting a mild blow to the chest. Others say it is painful and causes a forceful jerk. Any discomfort lasts only a moment but unless there are symptoms when the abnormal rhythm occurs, any shock(s) will be a surprise. Some patients are advised to avoid such things as working on a roof/tall ladder or swimming alone so if the ICD fires, they would be less likely to get hurt.

Remember your ICD will not make your heart any stronger. If you got tired easily or short of breath with exertion before ICD surgery, you will still have these symptoms afterward. If they occur, slow down or stop until the symptoms go away. Regular walking is encouraged for everyone and helps you get over the fatigue after surgery.

Special precautions:

Avoid intense magnetic fields (Ex: nuclear magnetic resonance imaging (NMRI), large magnets used in junk yards to move cars or magnets used to move hot steel in a smelting furnace.) These do not harm the ICD but can affect how they work. Some ICD's are turned off by a magnetic field and others are only temporarily affected. Let your doctor know if you ever hear "beeping tones" coming from your abdomen.

Stay an arm's length from the following electrical equipment since the signals can make it harder for the ICD to count your heart rate:

-large generators (as in factories, boats, or those which power a house) or power plants,
-high voltage power transformers and transmission lines,
-radio transmitters,
-walkie-talkie or radio control units for remote toys held within 6" of the pulse generator of the ICD, and
-arc welders.

The ICD pulse generator may trigger an alarm as you walk through a metal detector. No special precautions are needed when you pass through metal detectors of a public library or video store. However, advise airport security personnel before you walk through that you have an ICD and a "body search" is preferred to using the hand-held device over your ICD.

Diet/fluids:

Eat a healthy diet to regain your strength after ICD surgery. A low fat/low salt diet is best over the long-term to prevent other cardiac problems like fatty build-up in the blood vessels and high blood pressure. Keep your caffeine intake low in beverages (coffee, tea, colas) and foods (chocolate). As you may already know, caffeine can encourage abnormal heart rhythms.

Incision/Wound Care:

Most ICD incisions do not need any special cleaning after the patient is discharged from the hospital. Any crusts along the incision ("scabs") should be left alone - they will fall off in time. If there is no sign of infection, it is O.K. to have soap and water contact over the incision after 5 days. Be sure to finish taking the antibiotics as ordered to prevent infection.

Protect the area over the ICD pulse generator in your abdomen from sharp blows (rough-housing, tackle football, etc.). The soreness and any tendency of the ICD pulse generator to move when you turn over or first stand up will gradually go away over the next few weeks. Some patients get a loose binder from a medical supply house to provide gentle support to the pulse generator.

Problems to report to your doctor:

Problems are rare after ICD surgery, but be sure and call your doctor if you experience any of the following:

- signs of infection (redness, unusual warmth or swelling around the incisions, fever > 100 degrees, etc.)
- rapid heart beat or new spells of dizziness, fainting or weakness
- new soreness or fluid leaking from any of your incisions
- persistent cough or shortness of breath
- swelling of ankles, feet or hands

If your ICD fires once and you feel fine afterwards, telephone your doctor when it is convenient. Think back to see if there was anything that might explain your getting a shock such as forgetting a medication, unusual stress or fatigue, etc. If you get more than one shock in an hour, your doctor will probably advise that you go to the nearest emergency room. The nurses who do your ICD follow-up checks can be reached at _____ during usual office hours. Feel free to call them with any questions (or leave a message for them to call you back). If assistance is needed after hours, call _____ and the hospital operator will contact an electrophysiology doctor. A change in your medication may be needed. (Be assured that your doctor can use a special magnet over the ICD to keep the ICD from firing if needed).

Equipment/Supplies/Safety Aids

Community Resources (Agency & phone#):

Your ICD battery needs to be checked every couple of months. Although the life of an ICD battery varies depending on how much it is used, we expect most ICD batteries to last 3-5 years. Your first appointment is _____ in _____. Most of these checks will be 5-10 minute office visits where the ICD is "interrogated" (asked to report what has been going on). Other than these occasional ICD "check-ups," most health problems can be managed by your primary/local M.D.

We recommend that you keep the ICD identification card that we give you with you at all times. We also suggest that you get a Medic-Alert bracelet or necklace so anyone can find out about your ICD and medical condition by calling the 1-800 number listed on the metal tag. The nurse will give you the form to fill out before you leave the hospital.

Many patients enjoy meeting with other patients with an ICD! Although we care about your feelings and welcome any questions, sometimes the best advice comes from someone who has been through a similar experience. We will mail you an invitation to participate in our support group.

HEMODYNAMICS IN THE CARDIOTHORACIC INTENSIVE CARE UNIT: THE NURSING PROSPECTIVE

Mary Ellen Kern, R.N. M.S.N. C.C.R.N.

University of Medicine and Dentistry of New Jersey
Robert Wood Johnson Medical School
Cooper Hospital/University Medical Center
Camden, NJ

In the last twenty years, the delivery of healthcare at the bedside in the cardiothoracic intensive care unit (ICU) has become more complicated not only in terms of technology but also because of increased patient acuity, socioeconomic changes and constraints. The '80s and '90s have been marked by an increase in physiologic information and a multitude of options offered to the cardiothoracic surgical patient. This has certainly contributed to the complexity of issues now seen in the surgical suite and subsequently postoperatively in the cardiothoracic ICU. The cardiothoracic nurse is faced with an increased challenge in care which may vary according to the labor experience and educational background. Aside from achieving a level of comfort with the basic technical tasks of postoperative cardiothoracic care, the nurse is also challenged by the pharmacologic management and its integration with the hemodynamic status of the patient. The use of a wide variety of available vasoactive and hemodynamically responsive agents demands constant vigilance, reading and education on the part of those professionals who assume this awesome challenge in care. The integration of cardiopulmonary parameters and drug therapy offers the nurse an opportunity to optimize the patient's physiology on a moment-to-moment basis.

MONITORING CARDIOPULMONARY PARAMETERS

While the clinical picture of the patient is not solely indicated by measured hemodynamic parameters, they are helpful in determining patient response to certain therapies meant to optimize their cardiopulmonary status. These parameters most commonly include cardiac output, cardiac index, systemic vascular resistance (SVR), heart rate, mean arterial pressure (MAP), systolic/diastolic blood pressure, respiratory rate, arterial oxygen saturation (SaO_2), venous oxygen saturation (SvO_2), right atrial pressure (CVP), pulmonary artery pressure (PAP) and pulmonary artery occlusion pressure (PAOP).[1] Selectively, left atrial pressure, right ventricular pressure and pulmonary vascular resistance (PVR) are also utilized.[2] Most recently, SvO_2 and its reflection of tissue oxygenation related to applied therapies, the physiologic process of oxygen transport and its clinical outcome predictability has been studied.[3] The determinants of tissue oxygenation are cardiac output, hemoglobin concentration, the oxygen supply as well as the integrity of the structural and functional cellular and molecular complex. The balance between oxygen delivery (DO_2) and oxygen consumption (VO_2) which takes place within the cell is reflected by the SvO_2. Vasoactive substances such as epinephrine, which evoke the stress response may increase both, the myocardial, and systemic VO_2 resulting in a lower SvO_2. This triggers the need for more oxygen therapy, increased cardiac output, or more oxygen carrying capacity such as an increase in the hemoglobin level.

The determinants of cardiac output, i.e., heart rate and stroke volume (contractility, preload and afterload), may be manipulated by drug therapy. Oxygen administration may be followed by an attempt to increase the hemoglobin level, however, this is presently considered as the last resort due to a reluctance for blood product administration because of the risk of transmission of viral and bacterial infections. Other parameters, which may optimize cardiac output, such as fluid volume, are adjusted in conjunction with agents which enhance and preserve renal function.

Each category of vasoactive drug effects certain parameters, i.e., calcium antagonists effect heart rate and contractility, thus knowledge related to the titration of vasoactive substances becomes of utmost importance to the ICU nurse. If there is no prior history with a particular vasoactive substance, the administration of the drug should be carefully considered and monitored, since each patient demonstrates individual responses to any given therapy. Certain side-effects of FDA-approved drugs have been reported and related to a certain mechanism, and a scientific approach to the monitoring and documentation of all those outcome parameters which contribute to the clinical picture of the patient is important. Changes in drug dose should be followed up by sets of parameters to document the response. Essential to the proper assessment of the drug's contribution to a certain response is the patient's baseline hemodynamic profile prior to surgical intervention. Often, the catheterization report provides the patient's baseline values which may be used for future reference.

Although cardiac surgery often changes the quality of mechanical cardiac function, this change is over time and the baseline parameters still provide a basis for the evaluation of functional improvement or decline. It has been documented that hemodynamic values are related to the patient's age, i.e., after age 35, cardiac output decreases one percent per year.[4] At age 70, normal cardiac index is 2.5 L/min/m^2.[5]

Other elements such as the patient's sleep cycle are important information. Smolensky et al.[6] found that the patient's lowest cardiac output occurs during the patient's normal sleep time, while the peak cardiac output occurs at the middle of the patient's normal activity period. When illness, surgery and pharmacologic therapy are superimposed, the clinical picture becomes complicated. In this case, there may be a substantial difference in cardiac index between sleep and normal activity of up to 2 L/min/m^2.

CLASSIFICATION OF DRUGS AND THEIR HEMODYNAMIC RESPONSES

An understanding of the available commonly used agents in the vasoactive management of the postoperative cardiac surgical patient is briefly reviewed in this section.

Beta-blockers are negative inotropes which often decrease contractility.[7] Propranolol, esmolol and labetalol are examples of this category of drugs commonly used in the cardiothoracic ICU. When administered as a bolus, propranolol may be useful to control heart rate or hypertension. Esmolol and labetalol are usually administered as infusions. These agents require complete fluid resuscitation prior to drug administration in order to avoid hypotension. In such a case, tachycardia as a sign of dehydration, should be differentiated from true arrhythmia.[8]

Esmolol is metabolized in red blood cells and has a half-life of 2 minutes. It binds to plasma protein. Esmolol decreases heart rate, blood pressure, left ventricular ejection fraction (EF), and cardiac index. This drug potentiates digoxin (up to 20 percent increase in blood levels has been observed in normal volunteers). Because esmolol is cardioselective, it is relatively safe to use in patients with COPD or asthma. If needed, verapamil can be initiated within 20 minutes of discontinuation of esmolol. However, if treatment with verapamil has been initiated first, several hours need to elapse before esmolol can be safely started.[9] Labetalol has a different mechanism of action. The drug is a selective alpha-blocker and a non-selective beta-blocker. Used primarily for the treatment of hypertension and angina, labetalol increases cardiac and stroke index and decreases SVR and MAP. It inhibits reflex tachycardia. It is not recommended for patients with airway problems. The half-life of labetalol is 4 to 8 hours. Larsen and Larsen[10] reported the usefulness of labetalol in the treatment of epinephrine overdose.

Calcium channel blockers are a class of drugs which may be used to influence afterload by arterial dilation and contractility (negative inotropism) and preload by venous dilation.[7] Prototypes of this drug category are verapamil and diltiazem.[11]

Prostaglandins (PG) are a different class of substances. Alprostadil, (PGE$_1$), inhibits platelet aggregation and dilates blood vessels. The end-result is an increase in peripheral blood flow. The drug has a short half-life and is rapidly metabolized as 80 percent pass through the lungs. It has been widely used in neonates with congenital abnormalities and has only in the last ten years been used in adults for conditions ranging from baldness to impotency, to pulmonary hypertension.[12] Because of its short half-life, alprostadil is used as a continuous infusion. The hemodynamic effect is an increase in stroke volume and cardiac index. Reflex tachycardia and rise in body temperature with up to 3 degrees has been observed in some subjects.

Nitrates (nitroglycerine) are important drugs in cardiology for many postoperative cardiac surgical patients who require a controlled preload and coronary dilation to preserve graft flow. Usual dose is 50 to 100 µg/min.

Phosphodiesterase inhibitors (PDI) are a newer drug category with inotropic and vasodilating characteristics. Amrinone, milrinone and dopexamine are prototypes of PDI.

Amrinone has a half-life of 3 to 6 hours. It decreases VO_2 and, in this regard, is considered to be superior to dobutamine. It also increases cardiac index, EF and blood pressure and decreases left ventricular end-diastolic pressure (LVEDP).[13] It is considered to be synergistic with dobutamine and is useful in conjunction with dopamine and isoproterenol.[14] Amrinone also decreases afterload and improves contractility. This drug may cause thrombocytopenia.[15] Loading dose is 0.75 mg/kg and should be administered slowly over 3 minutes. The maintenance infusion rate is usually 5 to 30 µg/kg/min.

While milrinone has not been approved by the FDA for patients undergoing cardiac surgery, some studies have shown some therapeutic value in the postoperative cardiac surgical patient.[16,17] Milrinone is a derivative of amrinone which has a 20 time stronger inotropic action than amrinone. Its use usually results in increased heart rate, cardiac index, and left ventricular function. Milrinone generally decreases SVR, PVR, PAOP and LVEDP. The half-life is 1 to 2 hours and peaks in one hour.[18,19]

Dopexamine, an analogue of dopamine, is a newer drug. Its hemodynamic profile is presently under examination.[20] The applied principle is to preserve the dopamine-1 agonist properties while achieving afterload reduction with less direct positive inotropic effects.[21] It is 60 times more potent than dopamine.[20]

ALPHA- AND BETA-ADRENERGIC AGONISTS

Dopamine, first isolated in 1944, is a naturally occurring catecholamine with inotropic and vasopressor qualities.[22] It increases cardiac output, and systolic pressure but it has little effect on diastolic pressure. At low and intermediate doses, SVR remains unchanged. Its half-life is very short. It causes endogenous release of norepinephrine. It has a synergistic effect when used in conjunction with drugs such as nitroprusside, resulting in significantly enhanced left ventricular performance when compared with dopamine alone.[23]

Norepinephrine stimulates alpha and beta-1 receptors resulting in increased atrial and ventricular contractility. It also dilates the coronary arteries, increases venous return and the heart rate by enhancing ventricular conduction. It is considered a sympathomimetic hormone. Haft et al. reported that norepinephrine can cause catecholamine-induced platelet aggregation resulting in thrombosis of small vessels.[24]

Epinephrine, first isolated by Takamine and Aldrich in 1901, is a natural sympathomimetic hormone produced by the adrenal medulla.[25,26] It is still considered the most potent vasoconstrictor known to man. Because the drug suffers biodegradation in the presence of air and light, it is usually covered with a brown bag during administration.

In 1989, Roberts and Krisanda[27] reported an accidental intra-arterial injection of epinephrine during a cardiac arrest. While these types of accidents do not occur often, the potential for such mishaps should be considered during any code when a vasoconstricting agent is used, particularly in situations characterized by great anxiety when a patient arrests. This particular incident involved the injection of a preparation for immediate IV drug use. Epinephrine was injected and the limb became ischemic. Phentolamine was also administered through the same line to reverse the effect of epinephrine. Although the authors presented a successful, direct and apparently effective reversal of epinephrine, the response was unusual because generally, phentolamine is administered by subcutaneous infiltration.

Phenylephrine, synthesized in 1951, is an adrenergic stimulant which decreases cardiac output and heart rate and increases stroke volume and SVR with little effect on beta-receptors. It increases MAP, PAP and PAOP. Its half-life is 20 to 30 minutes. It is usually used to improve the hemodynamics in septic shock.[28]

Metaraminol is a positive inotrope and peripheral vasoconstrictor. Its rapid effect appears in 2 minutes. The drug has a half-life of 20 to 60 minutes. In combination with digoxin it may increase the ectopic arrhythmic activity. Its use has been beneficial in the treatment of cardiogenic shock.[29]

Dobutamine is a dopamine derivative first released in the United States in 1976. It is primarily used for the improvement of cardiac output and may increase heart rate at higher doses. It increases AV conduction and may result in rapid capture atrial fibrillation. The drug's onset of action is in 1 to 2 minutes and peaks at 10 minutes. Its half-life is 2 minutes. It is synergistic with nitroprusside and may be ineffective in patients receiving concomitant treatment with a beta-blocking agent. Usual starting dose is 5 µg/kg/min.[30]

Digoxin is a synthetic cardiotonic. The half-life is 36 hours after intravenous administration and is useful to improve contractility and cardiac output. In combination with beta-blockers, it may cause bradycardia and dysrhythmias, especially in patients with atrial fibrillation. Toxicity may occur if administered simultaneously with calcium preparations and furosemide. The loading dose should be based on ideal body weight (10 µg/kg).

Nitroprusside is a potent vasodilator which has a 30 second half-life. It decreases SVR thereby improving cardiac output. It has been shown to decrease platelet aggregation in some patients.

The choice of an agent like trimethaphan for control of afterload and hypertension should be considered in the postoperative phase of the cardiothoracic surgical patient especially in the presence of postoperative bleeding. Trimethaphan camsylate is a short acting ganglionic blocking agent which blocks acetylcholine at the receptor site and causes peripheral vasodilation. Diuretics, as well as the elevation of the head of the bed, may enhance the effect. This drug liberates histamine and should be used cautiously in the allergic patient.[31]

THE ADMINISTRATION AND WEANING OF VASOACTIVE SUBSTANCES

Each of the drugs briefly reviewed in this chapter effect particular hemodynamic parameters. The patients history, clinical assessment and the surgical course dictate which drugs can be weaned and which agents need to be maintained postoperatively until an oral preparation can be safely administered. Careful monitoring of the patient's response, sometimes on a moment-to-moment basis, and a clear understanding of the goals of therapy for any particular patient make the weaning of vasoactive substance a challenge. It is not uncommon to have a patient coming back from surgery on nitroglycerine for coronary protection, nitroprusside for afterload reduction, and dopamine, dobutamine or amrinone for improvement of cardiac output.

The process of weaning these drugs should begin with the drug which has the shortest half-life, since that is the drug most easily reversed if weaning fails. Moreover, the first drug to be weaned is the drug which has the highest potential for adverse effects. In either case, the nurse must consider that the patient needs time to adjust and respond to any change in therapy especially if the therapy has been administered for several days. This sometimes translates into reduction by a µg/hour or several hours depending on the patient's severity of disease. Drugs acting as neurotransmitters or hormones should be titrated slowly because the disease process may decrease the negative feedback response. It is important to emphasize that patient's survival depends upon the fragile titration of these drugs.

In order to demonstrate these principles, the following clinical scenario was developed:

> Mrs. H is a 54 year old woman post CABG x4 including right coronary artery (RCA), left anterior descending (LAD) and circumflex vessels. She returns to the ICU on 100 µg/min nitroglycerine. All parameters were repeated and all pertinent laboratory tests were ordered including arterial blood gas, electrolytes, CBC and coagulation profile. The following parameters are obtained: MAP 105 mm Hg, PAP 50/23 mm Hg, PAOP 23 mm Hg, RAP 18 mm Hg, cardiac output 3.2 L/min, CI 2.0 L/min/m^2, SVR 2175 dynes.sec/cm^5, SaO$_2$ 96%, SvO$_2$ 50%, hemoglobin 10 g/dL, Hct 30%, HR 100 beat/min.
>
> The patient is currently on 100 percent oxygen. Based on the above hemodynamic profile, it is decided that nitroglycerine should be continued for coronary protection, since the patient requires afterload reduction.
>
> After 30 minutes of treatment with nitroprusside, the following parameters were obtained: MAP 88 mm Hg, CO 4.5 L/min, PAP 40/15, CI 2.8 L/min/m^2, PAOP 15 mm Hg, SVR 1351 dynes.sec/cm^5, RAP 12 mm Hg, SvO$_2$ 65%.
>
> The patient is now a candidate for fluid resuscitation and further titration of nitroprusside. If the patient does not responded sufficiently to this trial of nitroprusside, other agents should be considered such as dobutamine or amrinone.

SUMMARY

The administration of pharmacologic agents in the postoperative period to achieve an optimal clinical picture is challenging and requires constant vigilance on the part of the nurse. This includes a sophisticated approach to the integration of hemodynamic values with the patient's baseline and current therapies. This is truly an ongoing challenge since there are always new technologies and therapies to be considered.

REFERENCES

1. White K: Using continuous SvO_2 to assess oxygen supply/demand balance in the critically ill patient. AACN Clinical Issues in Critical Care Nursing 1993;4(1):134–147.
2. Headley J, Diethorn M: Right ventricular volumetric monitoring. AACN Clinical Issues in Critical Care, 1993;4(1):120–133.
3. Ahrens T: Integration of hemodynamics and oxygenation. Trends in Critical Care, presentation, Philadelphia, PA, 1993.
4. Brandfonbrener M, Landowne M, Shock NW: Changes in cardiac output with age. Circulation, 1957;12:557.
5. Grossman W, Bain DS: Cardiac Catheterization Angiography and Intervention, 4th ed., Lea & Febinger, Philadelphia, PA, 1991.
6. Smolensky MH, Tatar SE, Bergman SA, et al: Circadian rhythmic aspect of human cardiovascular function: a review of chronobiologic statistical methods. Chronobiologia 1976;3:337–371.
7. Urban N: Hemodynamic clinical profiles. AACN Clinical Issues in Critical Care Nursing 1990;1:123.
8. Clark B: Beta adrenergic blocking agents: their current status. AACN Clinical Issues in Critical Care Nursing, 1992;3(2):447–460.
9. Blanski L, Lutz J, Laddu A: Esmolol, the first ultra-short-acting intravenous beta blocker for use in critically ill patients. Heart & Lung, 1988;17(1):80–89.
10. Larsen LS, Larsen A: Labetalol in the treatment of epinephrine overdose. Ann Emerg Med 1990;19:680–682.
11. White P: Calcium channel blockers. AACN Clinical Issues In Critical Care Nursing 1992;3(2):437–446.
12. D'Ambra MN, La Raia PJ, Philbin DM et al: Prostaglandin E_1. A new therapy for refractory right heart failure and pulmonary hypertension after mitral valve replacement. J Thorac Cardiovasc Surg 1985;89:567–572.
13. LeDoux, D: Management of heart failure in cardiac surgical patients: amrinone and other pharmacologic agents. Progress in Cardiovascular Nursing, 1990;5(3):78–83.
14. Goenen M, Pedemonte O, Baele P, Col J: Amrinone in the management of low cardiac output after open heart surgery. Am J Card 1985;56:33B-38B.
15. Gunnicker M, Hess W: Preliminary results with amrinone in perioperative low cardiac output syndrome. Thorac Cardiovasc Surg 1987;35:219–225.
16. Feneck RO: Effects of variable dose milrinone in patients with low cardiac output after cardiac surgery. Am Heart J 1991;121:1995–1999.
17. Wright EM, Sherry KM: Clinical and haemodynamic effects of milrinone in the treatment of low cardiac output after cardiac surgery. Br J Anaes 1991;67:585–590.
18. Baim DS, McDowell AV, Cherniles J, et al: Evaluation of a new bipyridine inotropic agent - milrinone in patients with severe congestive heart failure. N Engl J Med 1983;309:748–756.
19. Monrad ES, McKay RG, Baim DS, et al: Improvement in indexes of diastolic performance in patients with congestive heart failure treated with milrinone. Circulation 1984;70:1030–1037.
20. Smith GW, O'Connor SE: An introduction to the pharmacologic properties of Dopacard (dopexamine). Am J Cardiol 1988;62:9C-17C.
21. Gollub SB, Emmot WW, Johnson DE et al: Hemodynamic effects of dopexamine hydrochloride infusions of 48-72 hours duration for severe congestive heart failure. Am J Cardiology, 1988;62:83C-88C.
22. Watson: The isolation of dopamine. J Am Pharm Assoc 1944;33:270.
23. Miller CD, Stinson EB, Oyer PE, Derby GC, Reitz BA, Shumway NE: Postoperative enhancement of left ventricular performance by combined inotropic-vasodilator therapy with preload control. Thorac Cardiovasc Surg 1980;88:108.

24. Haft JI, Kranz PD, Albert FJ, et al: Intravascular platelet aggregation in the heart induced by norepinephrine: microscopic studies. Circulation 1972;46:698–707.
25. Takamine: Isolation of epinephrine from animal tissue. J Soc Chem Ind 1901;20:746.
26. Aldrich: Isolation of epinephrine. Am J Physiology 1901;5:547.
27. Roberts JR, Krisanda TJ: Accidental intra-arterial injection of epinephrine treated with phentolamine (letter) Ann Internal Med 1989;18:424–425.
28. Bergman and Sulzbacher: Synthesis of phenylephrine. J Organic Chemistry 1951;16:84.
29. Bourdarias JP, Dubourg O, Gueret P, et al: Inotropic agents in the treatment of cardiogenic shock. Pharmac Ther 1983;22:53–79.
30. Tright PV, Spray T, Pasque M, et al: The comparative effects of dopamine and dobutamine on ventricular mechanics after coronary artery bypass grafting: a pressure dimension analysis. Circulation 1984;70:I-112–117.
31. Corr L, Grounds RM, Brown MJ, et al: Plasma catecholamine changes during cardiopulmonary bypass: a randomized double blind comparison of trimethaphan camsylate and sodium nitroprusside. Br Heart J 1986;56:89–93.

FURTHER SUGGESTED BIBLIOGRAPHY

Clements J: Sympathomimetics, inotropics and vasodilators. AACN Clinical Issues in Critical Care Nursing, 1992(2):395–408.
Deglin J, Deglin S: Hypertension: current trends and choice in pharmacotherapeutics. AACN Clinical Issues in Critical Care Nursing, 1992;3(2):507–526.
Kelleher R, Rose A, Ordway L: Prostaglandins for the control of pulmonary hypertension in the postoperative cardiac surgery patient: nursing implications. Critical Care Nursing Clinics of North America, 1991;3(4):741–748.
Kuhn M: Nitrates. AACN Clinical Issues in Critical Care Nursing, 1992;3(2):409–422.
Woods S, Osguthorpe S: Cardiac output determinations. AACN Clinical Issues in Critical Care Nursing 1993;4(1):81–97.
Zaloga G, Prielipp R, Butterworth J, Royster R: Pharmacologic cardiovascular support. Critical Care Clinics 1993;9(2):335–362.

THORACIC AORTIC ANEURYSM ASSOCIATED WITH MARFAN SYNDROME

Jane V. Stewart, M.S.N., R.N., C.C.R.N.

Moorestown, New Jersey

OVERVIEW OF MARFAN SYNDROME

Marfan syndrome is a hereditary disorder of the connective tissue characterized by abnormally long extremities, arachnodactyly ocular malformations, bone and joint defects, and congenital cardiovascular anomalies. The disease was first identified by the French pediatrician Marfan in 1896. However, the medical world did not scrutinize this malady more extensively until the 1940's, when Etter and Glover began work on defining the bodily deformities associated with this disease.[1] McCusick further identified the cardiac abnormalities in the 1950's.[2] More recently, McCusick joined Pyeritz in looking at the molecular factors involved and have made further advances in the understanding of the disease process.[3]

Marfan syndrome is an autosomal dominant condition which is transmitted to approximately 50 percent of offspring. It is found in 1 in 21,000 live births. There seems to be no gender dominance. A defect in collagen formation is present leading to a cystic medial necrosis-like abnormality developed in the large arteries. Moreover, a fragmentation of the elastic fibers and mucoid deposition in the medial layer is present. This further results in a loss of elasticity and a weakening of the vessel wall.

MANIFESTATIONS OF MARFAN SYNDROME

The most common manifestations of this disease process are skeletal deformities, which are noted in 100 percent of afflicted patients. Ocular problems are present in 70 percent and cardiac, in as high as 80 percent. Skeletal manifestations commonly include a tall, lanky appearance with a short trunk and long arms. The arm span classically is greater than the patient's height. A positive *thumb* sign is also telltale evidence, when the length of the patient's thumb is so long it extends out laterally from his hand when it is folded over his palm. Sternal and spinal deformities may be noted as well, including pectus excavatum, pectus carinatum, scoliosis, and kyphosis. A narrow, highly arched palate may also be discovered on physical exam. These patients also exhibit very supple joints.

Ocular findings include lens subluxation, flattening of the cornea, and an increased globe length, which usually results in severe myopia. There is an increased chance of retinal detachments and an incidence of a bluish discoloration of the sclera in some patients.

Cardiac manifestations are by far the most problematic. Aortic aneurysm, dissection and rupture as well as insufficiency of the aortic and mitral valves associated with dysrhythmias are the most commonly reported manifestations. Annuloaortic ectasia, characterized by a greatly dilated aortic root, an enlarged ascending aorta, aortic valve incompetence, and cephalad displacement of the coronary arteries is most often described in these patients. It is usually seen in the aging patient, caused by years of wear and tear on these structures. But in the patient identified with Marfan syndrome, this is simply the final outcome of the disease process described earlier. Marfan syndrome accounts for the majority of dissecting aneurysms in persons under the age of 40. Dissection is the most common form of aneurysm and occurs, on average, at around 30 years of age. Unfortunately, the cardiac signs and symptoms often manifest themselves suddenly and without much warning.

MEDICAL DIAGNOSIS OF THORACIC ANEURYSM ASSOCIATED WITH MARFAN SYNDROME

Patients with Marfan syndrome present much the same way any acutely dissecting patient might. They will typically experience a sudden onset of dyspnea and/or angina which may be accompanied by a feeling of *doom.* Upon examination, unequal pulses, altered sensorium, tachycardia, tachypnea, and extreme restlessness may be noted. Rapid triage is a necessity as a major hemodynamic deterioration may occur in the patient. Chest roentgenograms, echocardiography, and aortography should be expected and preparation made by the nurses caring for these patients in the field, emergency department, or the critical care area.

The operating room team needs to be notified of the suspicious diagnosis while these patients are still undergoing aortography. This may allow to quickly assess resources and adequately prepare for surgical intervention. The goal of nursing care at this stage is to stabilize vital signs, support the patients and families emotionally, as well as educate them briefly in regard to the diagnosis, etiology, and plan of action over the next several hours. If surgery is indeed warranted, which is most likely will be, then the goal of preparing for surgery needs to be addressed.[4]

If an aortic aneurysm is confirmed, the major question for the surgeon is whether to repair it urgently or emergently. The answer to that really depends upon the type of aneurysm, its aortic location, and the state of the acute compromised cardiovascular perfusion. Typically, the surgeon will opt to work on attempting hemodynamic stabilization along with the cardiology and nursing teams, then elect for emergent repair sometime within the first twelve hours, (certainly within the first 24 hours). Emergent repair always carries with it a higher risk due to many factors, but is chosen often with this patient population due to the *sudden onset* nature of presentation and frequent rapid deterioration in cardiovascular parameters.

Operative repair may include varied approaches, but most often includes aortic valve replacement or repair, graft replacement of the ascending aorta, and possibly mitral valve repair or replacement. Aortic arch and descending aorta replacement may be necessary if these areas are affected. Any combination of these procedures may be utilized, depending upon the pathology present and surgeon preference.[4] Operative mortality in the presence of aortic rupture is generally above 50 percent. In the presence of dissection, it is known to be about 20 to 30 percent. In the case of aneurysm without dissection, a 5 to 10 percent mortality rate should be considered. There is an 80 to 90 percent five-year survival rate in patients with Marfan syndrome after surgical repair. Unfortunately, the 15-year survival rate is only 60 to 70 percent. These patients have a high incidence of recurrence of aneurysm due to the fact that the disease process is not stopped by surgical intervention.[1]

In Crawford's study of 43 patients with Marfan syndrome,[1] 14 had to return for second operations, five had to return a third time, and two had a fourth intervention. One patient had to have a sixth procedure done.

POSTOPERATIVE NURSING CONSIDERATIONS

Care for this patient population in the postoperative phase does not deviate much from the standard care of any other cardiac surgical patient.[5] The typical nursing plan of care includes addressing alterations in cardiovascular, pulmonary, gastrointestinal, urinary, thermoregulatory, and neurological systems in the immediate postoperative period. Many of these areas will continue to need attention as the patient moves toward discharge. Systemic arterial blood pressure should be carefully monitored, as problems would most definitely arise if it were to become elevated, even if only momentarily. It must be remembered that the great vessel walls are decidedly weakened in this disease state. Therefore, diligent care must be taken to avoid the labile pressure. Looking ahead toward discharge, nurses must also educate the patient and family members regarding the pathophysiology and compliance with ambulatory antihypertensive regimens.

HEREDITARY FACTORS AND FUTURE PREGNANCY

Since it is known that the Marfan syndrome trait is carried to approximately 50 percent of offspring, and that a person with Marfan's likely has a friable vascular system, it is not recommended that adult females with the disease consider having children, particularly since up to 51 percent of dissecting aortic aneurysms, in otherwise healthy women, under the age of 40, occurred during pregnancy. This may occur particularly because blood pressure and cardiac output are increased during pregnancy. Any female who has had repair of an existing aneurysm should also be warned that her oral anticoagulation regimen is teratogenic, further complicating an already risky prenatal picture. Genetic counseling and psychosocial intervention are appropriate avenues in the plan of care of the female patient with Marfan syndrome.

FOLLOW-UP CARE AND OTHER CONSIDERATIONS

Patients and family members will continue to need education and emotional support from the medical and nursing team after discharge from the hospital. Facts related to recurrence need to be carefully spelled out, together with encouragement of compliance with post-discharge medications and activity. It must be stressed that patients need to schedule and keep the recommended follow-up visits with the cardiologist. Blood pressure will be checked frequently, and echocardiography will be performed at regular intervals to look for recurrence of dilation. Surgeons typically recommend no further participation in contact sports or risky physical activities, due to the danger of rupture of a large vessel and bleeding from anticoagulation. Otherwise, patients undergoing repair for this disease may return to normal activity within the same time frame as those with other types of cardiac surgery.

Recent interest in this as well as other cardiac diseases among college and professional sports stars will most likely prompt further study of the causes and possible cures.[6] Until much more is understood and can be put to practical clinical use, the cardiothoracic team will still witness the most life-threatening manifestations of Marfan syndrome. Presently, the most life-saving technique available is surgical intervention.

REFERENCES

1. Crawford ES, Crawford JL: "Marfan's Syndrome" in diseases of the aorta. Williams and Wilkens, Baltimore, MD, 1984:215–47.
2. McCusick VA: The cardiovascular aspects of Marfan's Syndrome: A heritable disorder of connective tissue. Circulation 1955;11:321–42.
3. Pyeritz RE, McCusick VA: The Marfan Syndrome: diagnosis and management. N Engl J Med 1979;300:722–27.
4. Seifert PC: Dissecting aortic aneurysms. A problem in Marfan's syndrome. AORN J 1986;43(2):443–50.
5. Anderson JK: Marfan's syndrome. Crit Care Nurse 1991;11(4):69–72.
6. Vaska PL: Sudden cardiac death in young athletes: A review for nurses. AACN Clin Issues Crit Care Nurs 1992;3(1):243–54.

CONTROVERSIES IN THE MANAGEMENT OF THE CARDIAC SURGICAL PATIENT

Debra J. Lynn-McHale, M.S.N., R.N., C.C.R.N.

Thomas Jefferson University Hospital
Philadelphia, Pennsylvania

The last decade has been characterized by important advances in cardiac surgery techniques with great impact on cardiac surgical nursing. Along with these advances many controversies in patient care management have evolved. Such controversy usually involves treatment options as in the case of choosing treatment for patients with coronary artery disease (CAD). Medical management is applied initially to many patients with cardiac symptoms. Effective treatment may be achieved with beta-blockers, calcium-channel blockers, and/or nitrates. Other treatment options include percutaneous transluminal coronary angioplasty (PTCA), placement of stents, atherectomy, and laser therapy. Unfortunately, restenosis is a significant problem with rates ranging from 30 to 50 percent depending on the therapy. Another treatment option for patients with CAD is coronary artery bypass graft surgery.

Although a variety of treatment options exist for patients with CAD it is not clear which is the most effective long-term. Initially, it was thought that the use of interventional therapies would decrease the necessity for cardiac surgery. That has not proven to be true. In reality, the use of interventional therapies may only delay the need of cardiac surgery. Future outcome studies will determine the most appropriate treatment options.

Cardiac surgery should lengthen life and enhance the quality of life. Several studies have investigated the effects of cardiac surgery and its impact on increasing life expectancy.[1] The European Coronary Surgery Study found a 73 percent survival rate in patients who were medically managed, and a 91 percent survival rate in those who were surgically treated.[2] Another study[3], reported the long-term (eight years) follow-up of CAD patients treated medically and surgically. This study found a 25 percent increase in survival for patients treated surgically versus those treated medically. To date, there are few long-term studies comparing patients treated with interventional therapy versus cardiac surgery. These data are essential for future decision making regarding treatment options. Controversy advances in cardiac surgery exists in determining which grafts work best for bypassing occluded coronary arteries. Saphenous veins have been used extensively, yet data on saphenous vein graft patency 1 year post surgery is 76 percent and at 10 years is 52 percent.[4,5] Internal mammary arteries have shown great promise and have been utilized successfully for cardiac bypass surgery. Internal mammary arteries demonstrate 85 to 95 percent patency 7 to 10 years post cardiac surgery.[6] The gastroepiploic artery has also been used for coronary bypass. It is a large artery positioned along the greater curvature of the stomach. It is usually used to bypass the posterior, circumflex, or right coronary arteries. Data have shown good early patency rates, however, it is premature to assess the long-term results. The inferior epigastric artery was first used in 1988. It is generally used as a free graft. Early patency data is not yet available. Other grafts used for coronary artery bypass include the cephalic artery, internal mammary vein, internal thoracic artery, radial artery, and the splenic artery. It is possible that additional conduits will be added to the list in the future as the debate as to which is the best bypass graft continues. Presently, the internal mammary artery is recommended as the conduit of choice for its increased long-term patency rate.

Treatment of valvular disease is still controversial. Valve surgery is indicated when medical management does not alleviate symptoms of cardiac dysfunction. An important question is whether the natural valve should be repaired or replaced. Valve repair include open mitral commissurotomy, annuloplasty, and valve leaflet reconstruction. Although currently under debate, it is thought that the valve should be repaired, if possible, instead of being replaced, as the repair of the patient's native valve promotes the best hemodynamic functioning and prevents or delays the need for a valve replacement. Many centers are presently repairing mitral valves, while others are also repairing aortic valves. From the technical point of view, the valve repair may be more difficult to accomplish, thus increasing the patient's time on cardiopulmonary bypass and the length of anesthesia. It is essential that the surgeon assess the risks/benefits of valve repair versus replacement.

Choosing the best valve to insert for those who need valve replacement is essential. With over 50 types of prosthetic valves on the market, surgeons are often faced with a difficult decision. Various mechanical and biological valves are available. Factors that need to be considered when selecting a prosthetic valve include the patient's age, activity status, and the ability to take anticoagulants. Controversy may exist when determining what valve should be inserted in which patient, and what criteria should be used in the process. Controversy also exists as to which valve is the most effective for specific patients and disorders.

PERIOPERATIVE ISSUES

A new trend for many health care centers is same day admission for cardiac surgery. Not all centers have coordinated this admission option. Many institutions continue to prefer to admit patients the evening prior to surgery. Same day admission is one strategy hospitals have employed to decrease the length of stay.

Family liaison nurses are available in many centers. The liaison nurse keeps family members informed of the patients progress as they wait during cardiac surgery. Controversy often exists regarding the value of such a position. There is evidence which supports the importance of keeping family updated, as it can facilitate family coping. Even if the patient is not doing well in the operating room, the family can begin to mobilize necessary resources.

There is much debate regarding myocardial protection during cardiac surgery. This includes the use of warm versus cold cardioplegia, as well as the use of antegrade and retrograde perfusion. Cold cardioplegia decreases cellular metabolism in an effort to preserve the myocardium. Cold cardioplegia can cause myocardial depression, and warm cardioplegia has been advocated and used in some centers in an effort to eliminate potential problems related to the use of cold cardioplegia. Additional research is needed to help practitioners select the most effective temperature of cardioplegia solutions.

Another controversy involves the administration of cardioplegia, i.e., the use of antegrade versus retrograde perfusion. Antegrade delivery of cardioplegia, via the coronary ostia, has traditionally been used to assist with myocardial cooling. Currently, retrograde perfusion is being used by more centers. Retrograde perfusion, involves the administration of cardioplegia solution into the coronary sinus through the coronary veins, thus providing a *back door* approach to myocardial protection. Retrograde cardioplegia may be used in conjunction with antegrade perfusion, in an effort to offer additional myocardial protection. Again, more studies are necessary to determine which method or combination of methods are most effective.

Controversy also exists regarding several techniques used in the postoperative period. One such issue is the management of postoperative hypothermia. In the past, the patient came to the intensive care unit from the operating room quite cold and achieved normothermia, gradually without intervention. Currently, rewarming is thought to be the most effective way to improve homeostasis. Rewarming is initiated in the operating room and continues in the intensive care unit. There are a variety of rewarming mechanisms which include warmed oxygen, infrared lamps, covering the patient's head, thermal blankets, warmed IV solution, conductive air mattresses and radiant heat devices. Howell et al.[7] studied the use of different head coverings and patient rewarming techniques post-cardiac surgery and found no significant difference in patient rewarming rates. Oliver and Fuessel[8] studied the use of three different warming techniques on patients post cardiac surgery. They found no statistical difference in rewarming patients using normal blankets, warmed blankets, or electric blankets. Additional research is needed to determine the most effective method for patient rewarming.

Assessment and treatment of postoperative shivering varies greatly from center to center. Holtzchaw[9] recommends the use of a shivering assessment tool which provides an objective way to increase the degree of patient shivering. SvO_2 monitoring has been useful to demonstrate changes in oxygen consumption. Shivering increases heart rate, metabolic needs, carbon dioxide production, increases myocardial workload, and depresses myocardial contractility. Pharmacological treatment for shivering includes administration of demerol and morphine sulfate. Since shivering may have detrimental effects, its accurate assessment and treatment is of utmost importance.

Postoperative fluid replacement can often be challenging. Controversy exists regarding the use of crystalloids versus colloids. Crystalloids tend to leak into the interstitial space, thus only a small amount actually remains intravascularly. If one liter of crystalloid is administered, approximately 80 percent of it will leak into the interstitial tissue, and the other 20 percent will remain in the intravascular space.[10] The administration of colloids may allow a larger quantity of fluid to remain in the intravascular space. Colloid administration may increase the oncotic pressure and facilitate the movement of fluid from the interstitial space into the intravascular space. Moreover, the presence of vasoactive substances released post bypass surgery may potentiate the transfer of colloids and other fluids out into the interstitial space.

One question often asked is "are postoperative weights necessary in the critical care setting?" Many, now say, no. Although weights were routinely part of the data collected for assessment of fluid therapy, many now believe it is not necessary. Using a sling type scale often greatly increases patient oxygen consumption and patient discomfort. Intake and output, pulmonary artery parameters, and lung sounds are reliable indices of fluid status. Since the majority of cardiac surgical patients are ambulating by postoperative day two, they can easily be weighed on a stand-up scale. Daily weights can be obtained and compared to weights prior to discharge.

Minimizing postoperative bleeding is increasingly important. Effective management of mediastinal chest tubes is one mechanism for achieving this objective. Maintaining chest tube patency is essential. Milking versus stripping chest tubes remains controversial. Milking involves fan-folding the chest tube and gently compressing the tubing. This creates a pressure gradient of approximately -50 cm H_2O. Stripping (whether by hand or using mechanical devices) can create a pressure gradient up to -400 cm H_2O.[11] Although milking is the preferred technique, it should be performed only as necessary. Milking is usually effective in breaking up most thrombi and maintaining chest tube patency. Stripping should only be used as a last resort in an attempt to remove extensive clots and prevent tamponade.

Another method to minimize postoperative bleeding is to prevent or control hypertension. It is ideal to maintain the patient's mean arterial pressure between 65 to 70 mm Hg,[12] especially the first 8 to 12 hours post surgery. This is often achieved with vasodilator therapy. Reducing the patient's blood pressure, will decrease stress on the newly bypassed graft suture lines.

Positive end-expiratory pressure (PEEP) may also be used in an effort to decrease postoperative bleeding. The increase in intrathoracic pressure produced by PEEP may compress small cardiac vessels, thus decreasing bleeding. There is little scientific data to support this theory, yet anecdotally practice has demonstrated that it often works.

Pharmacological manipulation of intra- and postoperative bleeding may be necessary. Many options are available including protamine sulfate, epsilon aminocaproic acid, desmopressin, and aprotinin. Since some of these therapies are expensive, judicious use of these products is essential.

Blood and blood component therapy may also be necessary for patients during or after cardiac surgery. Patients with a hematocrit below 30% or hemoglobin below 8 g/dL may require transfusion. Other centers may use values as low as a hematocrit below 20% and a hemoglobin level below 6 g/dL as transfusion trigger. A trend toward lower hematocrit and hemoglobin levels prior to transfusion is evident, even in the elderly. Zeler et al.[13] compared the efficacy of a protocol devised by critical care nurses for managing postoperative cardiac surgery bleeding to traditional management. The critical care nurses performed bedside activated clotting time (ACT) testing, managed chest tube drainage, and determined when autotransfusion and blood replacement were needed. The study demonstrated a decrease in blood loss (mean 150 cc/patient), decreased use of replacement therapy, and decreased occurrence of reoperations for postoperative bleeding.

There are a variety of devices currently on the market for hemodynamic monitoring. The most controversial are the pulmonary artery catheters which are able to measure pressures, volumes, mixed venous oxygen saturation (SvO_2), ejection fraction, and continuous cardiac output. Choosing which catheter to insert is often difficult. Pulmonary artery catheters provide accurate data regarding pulmonary artery pressures and pulmonary artery occlusion pressure, thus eliminating the need for left atrial catheters and the potential risks that are associated with their use.

SvO_2 monitoring has played a major role in patient management post cardiac surgery. It is beneficial in providing data regarding patient response to titration of vasoactive agents. It also provides useful data during patient suctioning. A sharp decrease in SvO_2 provides indication for a change in suctioning strategies. SvO_2 data can also provide guidance regarding changes in patient position, as the patient may tolerate one side better than the other. The use of SvO_2 monitoring is very controversial, particularly when the additional catheter cost is considered. SvO_2 values greater than 65 percent post cardiac surgery have been associated with fewer postoperative complications, whereas consistently low SvO_2 values, ranging between 40 and 60 percent were associated with increased mortality and morbidity.[14]

In addition to pulmonary artery pressures, the right heart catheter (Baxter Healthcare Corp., Irvine, CA) provides data regarding right heart volumes and an estimate of right ventricular ejection fraction. It is not yet conclusive if there is a direct correlation between cardiac volumes and pressures. This may be particularly true in patients experiencing cardiac tamponade.

The ability to obtain continuous measurement of cardiac output has been added to some pulmonary artery catheters. A digital cardiac output value is updated on the monitor every 30 seconds. This promising technology, may not only provide essential hemodynamic data, but also significantly decrease the time spent obtaining cardiac output, thus increasing the time critical care nurses may dedicate for other patient care needs.

Although there are significant advances in pulmonary artery catheter technology, it is yet to be determined its exact impact on patient's outcome. Some centers are no longer inserting pulmonary artery catheters for routine cardiac operations but are using central line catheters instead. The future will continue to challenge the health care providers to examine their practice and select the most appropriate strategies for the cardiac surgical patients.

REFERENCES

1. Lembo N, King S: Randomized trials of percutaneous transluminal coronary angioplasty, coronary artery bypass grafting, or medical therapy in patients with coronary artery disease. Cor Art Dis 1990;1:449–454.
2. European Coronary Surgery Study Group: Prospective randomized study of coronary artery bypass surgery in stable angina pectoris. Second interim report by the coronary surgery study group. Lancet 1980;2:491–495.
3. CASS Principle Investigators and their Associates: Coronary artery surgery study (CASS): A randomized trial of coronary artery bypass surgery. Survival data. Circulation 1983;68:939–950.
4. Grondin C, Campeau L, Lesperance J, Enjolbert M, Bourassa M: Comparison of late changes in internal mammary artery and saphenous vein grafts in two consecutive series of patients 10 years after operation. Circulation 1984;70(suppl. 1):I208-I212.
5. Lytle B, Loop F, Cosgrove D, Ratliff N, Easley K, Taylor P: Long term serial studies of internal mammary artery and saphenous vein coronary bypass grafts. J Thorac Cardiovasc Surg 1985;89:248–258.
6. Loop FD, Lytle BW, Cosgrove DM, et al: Influence of the internal-mammary-artery graft on 10-year survival and other cardiac events. N Eng J Med 1986;314:1–6.
7. Howell RD, Dawn L, Sanjines S, Burke J, DeStefano P: Effects of two types of head coverings in the rewarming of patients after coronary artery bypass graft surgery. Heart & Lung 1992;21:1–5.
8. Oliver SK, Fuessel E: Control of postoperative hypothermia in cardiovascular surgery patients. Crit Care Nurs Quarterly 1990;12:63–68.
9. Holtzchaw BJ: Postoperative shivering after cardiac surgery: a review. Heart & Lung 1985;15:292–300.
10. Norris SO: Managing low cardiac output states: maintaining volume after cardiac surgery. AACN Clinical Issues in Critical Care Nursing 1993;4:309–319.
11. Duncan D, Erickson R: Pressures associated with chest tube stripping. Heart & Lung 1982;11:166–171.
12. Brown MM, Kemper KM: Control of postoperative bleeding in the cardiac surgery patient. J Cardiovasc Nurs 1993;7:59–70.
13. Zeler KM, McPharlane TJ, Salamonsen RJ: Effectiveness of nursing involvement in bedside monitoring and control of coagulation status after cardiac surgery. Am J Crit Care 1992;1:70–75.
14. Krauss XH, Verdou PD, Hugenholtz PG, Navta J: On-line monitoring of mixed venous oxygen saturation after cardiothoracic surgery. Thorax 1975;30:636–43.

REHABILITATION POST CARDIAC SURGERY

Susan G. Burrows, R.N., M.N.

Emory University Hospital
Atlanta, GA

Heart disease continues to be the number one cause of death in the United States. Approximately 94.5 billion dollars are spent on the diagnosis, treatment and procedures associated with cardiovascular illness. Approximately one-third of all these procedures are performed on patients over age 65.[1] With the tremendous advances in technology, population continues to age. It is estimated that by the year 2010, one in five Americans will be over 65. The implication for the financial impact on our economy is astounding. Cardiac surgery is being closely scrutinized by consumers and third-party payors regarding costs, delivery systems, approaches and outcomes. Terms such as cost-containment, streamlining, fast-tracking, managed care, re-engineering care and clinical pathways are becoming familiar to nurses involved with cardiac surgery patients. Tremendous pressures for cost-effective, quality outcomes are key factors driving the changes in the delivery of health care.

Coronary artery bypass surgery is listed as the most expensive commonly performed surgery and thus has received a lot of attention. The success of aggressive recovery post-bypass surgery rests on re-engineering postoperative care and radically reducing both, critical care stay and overall length of stay. In a recent review,[2] a protocol for fast-track coronary bypass surgery (CABG) was outlined. This protocol, which may significantly reduce hospital stay, emphasizes preoperative education, administration of certain medications and accelerated program for extubation and activity. Clearly, the viability of cardiac programs in the 1990's rests on being able to provide cost-effective, quality care.

At Emory University Hospital, a CABG Clinical Path was initiated March 15, 1993, and by May 15, 1993, the hospital length of stay had already been reduced by two days. The Clinical Path was developed by a multi-disciplinary team committed to re-thinking our delivery of care and to challenging our own paradigms. We defined optimal time lines for sequencing procedures and interventions and began to look critically at outcomes. We questioned the reason for patients not meeting an expected outcome. *Why wasn't the patient extubated and transferred to the telemetry floor within 24 hours? How can we achieve an accelerated activity schedule? How can we provide a comprehensive education program for patients discharged 4 to 5 days postoperatively? What survival skills must be learned prior to discharge and what is in place to provide the information and skills needed after discharge?*

In addition to the pressures of reducing the length of stay, cutting costs and improving quality, health care providers are also faced with the reality that the types of patients that undergo cardiac surgery are older, sicker and more complex. They are admitted the evening before or increasingly more often the day of surgery. The time to prepare the patient and the family is compressed. For many, the time from the initial cardiac event to catheterization, surgery and discharge is so rapid that it is difficult for them to comprehend even the extent of their illness. Nurses have a unique opportunity to positively impact the quality of care and reduce the length of stay, as they gain expertise in technological and bio-behavioral techniques. Nurses can provide a healing environment rather than a disease-management environment. Promotion of health as well as prevention of illness can be emphasized, helping people to develop the skills and commitment to maintain wellness. Nurses are a vital resource in the rehabilitation process.

The definition of *rehabilitation* is *to restore to a former capacity and to bring to a condition of health or useful and constructive activity*. Cardiac rehabilitation programs help patients regain physical and psychological abilities so they may return to functional and productive lives.[3] Cardiac rehabilitation is a continuous process that has arbitrarily been divided into three phases. Phase I usually begins within 24 to 48 hours after the event and continues until the patient is discharged. Phase II is a supervised, planned cardiac rehabilitation program that begins after discharge and lasts 10 to 12 weeks. Phase III is the life-long program.[3]

Goals during Phase I include physical reconditioning, education of the patient and the family including, coping skills and psychological support during the early recovery phase. Patients who are extubated on the day of surgery or within 12 to 14 hours post procedure may be transferred to a telemetry unit within 24 hours. Adequate pain management, early removal of chest tubes, aggressive pulmonary toilet and accelerated activity schedules can dramatically impact a patient's progression.

It is important to emphasize the role of adequate pain management. Typically, at the end of the first or second postoperative day, patients may move more, however, they often do not express the full extent of their pain. Pain may contribute to delay early ambulation and patients may not be able or eager to accept and attribute it to their discomfort. Generally, there is a tendency to under medicate patients. The patient's comfort is correlated to the level of aggressiveness of activity and treatments.

Deconditioning occurs very quickly. Studies have shown that it takes approximately 24 hours of bed rest for the body to begin to decondition[3] which is characterized by muscle atrophy, loss of joint flexibility and reduction in vital capacity and lung volumes/ In addition, decreased venous tone and venous return can deplete intravascular volume and cause postural hypotension and tachycardia. As little as three hours of daily upright posture can diminish the de-conditioning effects of bed rest.[3]

The patient's activity increases gradually from sitting in the chair, up to the bathroom, walking in the room, to walking the halls. Endurance is increased with frequent short walks as opposed to long exhausting walks. Clinical assessment including heart rate, rhythm, blood pressure, arterial oxygen saturation and level of fatigue (dyspnea) determines progression. Pulse oximetry can be used to wean patients from oxygen therapy and to further evaluate ambulatory status with and without oxygen administration. The systolic blood pressure should rise with exercise and the diastolic should remain at the same level or decrease slightly. If the systolic arterial pressure falls more than 15 mm Hg or the diastolic pressure rises more than 10 mm Hg, cessation and re-evaluation is necessary. The Borg Scale of Rate of Perceived Exertion (RPE) is a useful tool for monitoring exercise. This scale gives a numerical value to a perceived level of exertion. The scale was developed by determining heart rates of healthy people and correlating their subjective response to different levels of exercise. Patients should walk or exercise at an RPE of 11 to 15. They identify which number (from 6 to 20) best describes how they feel and adjust as needed.[4] Walking specific distances and having *distance or check points* posted in the hallways has also been suggested. One can compute a target heart rate by adding 20 beats to the resting pulse at an RPE less than 14.

Supervising ambulation provides the nurse with an opportunity to reinforce with the patient that "overdoing" will not damage his/her heart, explain the deconditioning process, as well as ways of improving strength and endurance. The patient should be encouraged to look closely at his daily progress and not the total, long-term picture. *Was it easier for him to shave or bathe today as compared to yesterday? Was it easier and more comfortable getting out of bed today?*

Patient and family education is an ongoing, dynamic and essential component of the recovery process. The crises of hospitalization and surgery, in addition to the anesthesia, pain, sleep deprivation, anemia, fatigue and medications create major barriers to learning. Comprehension and retention are minimal. Since attention span and memory are limited, short repetitive teaching sessions are more beneficial. The immediate physiological and safety needs are priority. Patients feel vulnerable and overwhelmed. They are less interested in knowing why events occur and more in how to survive them. Education needs to be focused on reducing the unknown and providing information so that new experiences are more predictable and familiar.

Preoperatively, patients should be informed about what to expect from their surgery, routine ICU procedures, and expectations during the postoperative recovery. This information is frequently given on an outpatient basis, in the physician's office or the evening before surgery. Depending on the time when this information is provided, it can either add to, or reduce the anxiety associated with surgery. Preoperative counseling is the key to moving patients along, but attention should be paid to not having them feel they are on an assembly line. Written and visual materials are essential in reinforcing content and providing a resource for future reference.

The primary teaching goals for the preoperative period are: 1) to reduce anxiety by providing an overview of the entire process; 2) to elicit cooperation and participation regarding postoperative activity progression; and 3) to achieve competency in postoperative respiratory exercises.

Patients who understand the clinical benefits of an aggressive recovery program will have a more positive attitude about possible discharge on the third, fourth or fifth postoperative day.

Facing the reality of a reduced length of hospital stay, increased patient age and complex problems, there is much debate on *how*, *when* and *what* should be taught in the hospital. Numerous studies on cardiac patients performed in the 1980's designed to identify patient's informational needs, looked at the timing when the information was provided and how this information was retained. At that time, it was felt that patients were given too much too soon. On the other hand, in a recent study by Hanisch,[5] patients post myocardial infarction and CABG were asked to rate the importance of 30 specific informational items related to cardiac education. Respondents believed that the majority of items should be taught after the event but prior to discharge and then later reinforced.

Research related to the educational needs of patients in the 90's will help us better define and redesign our cardiac programs. The challenge is to provide information to the patient and influence behavior in such a way that attitudes and actions will be focused on improving and maintaining health. It is important to prepare patients to make informed choices. Ideally, a partnership should be established with the patients honoring their values and attitudes inherent in their decision making. Attitudes of power and control that suggest the patient must follow healthcare providers' dictates because "they know best" will probably not be successful in the long-run. Even the word *compliance* is somewhat outdated. Terms such as *adherence*, *cooperation* or *concurrence* suggest choice and mutuality of goals.

It is important to maximize the time spent with patients and families in the postoperative period. At Emory, they receive a discharge book as soon as they are transferred to the floor. The families often start reading the material immediately.[6] Information such as risk factor modification, activity progression, medication precautions and wound care can be shared by the nurse during routine care activities. This information is reinforced with written and visual materials. The *formal* patient/family conference is scheduled prior to discharge. Emphasis should be placed on the importance of smoking cessation, progressing activity, improved strength and endurance, precautions related to sternal healing and problems to report after discharge.[6]

Prior to discharge, one should begin to lay a foundation regarding patient's diet, exercise, risk factor modification and stress management. Although many healthcare providers are knowledgeable about the physiologic benefits of relaxation, visualization and meditation, not many of them routinely practice these with their patients. Teaching patients to relax can improve sleep patterns, reduce medication requirements and provide a more peaceful, psychological balanced state. Patients may also be more receptive to other suggestions for recovery.[7]

The entry into a phase II cardiac rehabilitation program within 1 to 2 weeks post discharge may facilitate a more rapid overall recovery and return to optimal state of health. In 1987, the Public Health Service Report[8] concluded that, " .... rehabilitation programs are safe, and effectively increase the functional capacity of patients who have had myocardial infarction (MI), CABG or have stable angina." The Health Care Financing Administration (HCFA) has used these recommendations for coverage policy decisions for Medicare. It also seems likely that the new health care reform will include an added focus on patient education, prevention and early intervention as a means of reducing health care costs.

The phase II program is a supervised, planned cardiac rehab program that usually lasts 10 to 12 weeks. The first two-week sessions are monitored. This may vary according to the individual patient's condition. According to the American Heart Association on Exercise Standards, an activity classification was established to provide guidelines for activity, monitoring and supervision for various conditions (Table 1).[9]

Contraindications to exercise include symptoms of angina, hypotension, heart failure and uncontrolled dysrhythmias.

Exercise testing for rehabilitation is recommended before a training program has actually begun. The exercise prescription and protocols must be individualized to each patient. At the Emory Health Enhancement Program (EHEP), entry into phase II begins with exercise testing and determination of oxygen consumption. Peak oxygen consumption is the maximum amount of oxygen the body can extract and use from inspired air during exercise testing. The percent of maximum oxygen consumption helps determine the frequency, duration, intensity and progression of exercise.[10]

The electrocardiographic and hemodynamic responses, along with the subjective responses and the patient's response to perceived rate of exertion (Borg scale) are also evaluated. Typically, the prescribed workloads yield approximately 50 percent of that individuals target heart rate range. Various tables and protocols are then used as guides for prescribing metabolic equivalent of a task (MET) levels. The MET is a common way to measure the workload of various activities on the cardiopulmonary system. One MET is the amount of oxygen expended in the resting state (3.5 mL/kg/min).[10] An activity such as walking 3 mph that requires four times the resting metabolic demand, is quantitated at the 4 MET level. The MET remains the same as long as the speed or the difficulty of the workout remains at the same level.

The exercise prescriptions are individualized, i.e., the 75 year old CABG patient, the 50 year old with an ejection fraction of 30 percent and the 40 year old with a 26% hematocrit will probably be at different levels. As they progress, they will be re-evaluated and prescriptions redefined.

Patient/family education, coaching and counseling is also a vital component of a successful rehabilitation program. A multi-disciplinary team should work with the patient to provide new information, reinforce hospital teaching, clarify misconceptions and provide an atmosphere in which the patient can make informed choices about his/her health care.

Risk factor modification can result in slowing and possible reversal of disease. When admitted to the hospital, patients who have just ceased smoking may need tremendous support, encouragement and intervention following discharge. Smoking is an addiction, and healthcare providers' attitude must not be one of righteous indignation. Clear, factual information regarding the dangers of smoking should be provided. The incidence of reinfarction and death is twice as high for those who continue to smoke. Smoking causes increased platelet aggregation and coronary spasm. Data related to the effects of smoking on the coronary patient, should be presented.[3] Patients must be educated to recognize high-risk behaviors, situations and strategies for intervention, and stress management tech-

Table 1. Recommendations of the American Heart Association on Exercise Standards

Activity Classification	Clinical Characteristics	Activity Guidelines
Class A	Apparently healthy, under age 40, no evidence of increased risk for exercise, no symptoms of or known presence of heart disease or major risk markers, individuals of any age without known heart disease or major risk markers and who have a normal exercise test.	No restrictions other than basic guidelines. ECG, blood pressure monitoring and supervision not required.
Class B	Presence of known, stable cardiovascular disease with low risk for vigorous exercise. Includes individuals with CAD, post MI, CABG, PTCA, angina pectoris, abnormal exercise test and abnormal coronary angiograms or with valvular heart disease, congenital heart disease, cardiomyopathy and with exercise test abnormalities that do not meet the criteria outlined in C and D below. NYHA class 1 or 2, exercise capacity over 6 MET, no evidence of heart failure, free of ischemia or angina at rest or on the exercise test at or below 6 MET, appropriate rise in systolic blood pressure during exercise, no sequential premature ventricular contractions and the ability to satisfactorily self-monitor intensity of activity.	Activity should be individualized with exercise prescription by qualified personnel or restricted to walking, ECG and blood pressure monitoring during prescription procedures, medical supervision required during prescription sessions and nonmedical supervision for other exercise sessions if the individual understands how to monitor his/her activities.
Class C	Same as class B, except unable to self-regulate or to understand recommended activity levels.	Same as class B with supervision by nonmedical personnel trained in basic CPR or with electronic monitoring at home.
Class D	Those at moderate to high risk for cardiac complications during exercise including individuals with CAD, cardiomyopathy, valvular heart disease, exercise test abnormalities not directly related to ischemia, previous episode of ventricular fibrillation or cardiac arrest that did not occur in the presence of an acute ischemic event or cardiac procedure, patients with complex ventricular arrhythmias that are uncontrolled at mild to moderate work intensities with medication, individuals with three-vessel disease or left main disease and individuals with low ejection fractions (less than 30%), two or more MIs, NYHA class 3 or greater, exercise capacity less than 6 MET, ischemic horizontal or downsloping ST depression of 4.0 mm or more or angina during exercise, fall in systolic blood pressure with exercise, a medical problem that may be life-threatening, previous episode of primary cardiac arrest and ventricular tachycardia at a work load of less than 6 MET.	Activity should be individualized with exercise prescription by qualified personnel. ECG, blood pressure monitoring and medical supervision should be continuous during rehabilitation sessions until safety is established (usually 6 to 12 sessions or more).
Class E	Unstable disease with activity restrictions including individuals with unstable ischemia, heart failure that is not compensated, uncontrolled arrhythmias, severe and symptomatic aortic stenosis and other conditions that could be aggravated by exercise.	No activity is recommended for conditioning purposes. Attention should be directed to treating the patient and restoring him/her to class D or higher. Daily activities must be prescribed based on individual assessment by the patient's personal physician.

Adapted from: AHA Exercise Standards. Circulation 1990;82(6):2308-09.

niques. Moreover, if needed, they should be encouraged to participate in formal programs for smoking cessation.

An elevated cholesterol level is a major risk factor for the cardiac surgical patient. Dietary intervention directed towards lowering total fat, saturated fat and cholesterol and achieving ideal weight can usually make a significant impact.[11] Acceptable blood level for total cholesterol is less than 200 mg/dL, for HDL equal to 60 mg/dL or greater and for LDL less than or equal to 130 mg/dL. An HDL of 35 mg/dL or less is considered a major risk factor. The dietary recommendation for the general public is to have 30 percent or less of the daily calories from total fat and no more than 8 to 10 percent of these calories derived from saturated fat.[12] Patients with coronary disease should have less than 200 mg/dL cholesterol and less than 7 percent saturated fat per day. It should be emphasized that modification of this risk factor is much too complicated, even for today's weight-conscious society. Not many people know the number of calories ingested daily, or how to accurately calculate the percentage of total and/or saturated fat. Terms such as polyunsaturated, monounsaturated, and hydrogenated fat should be carefully explained. Sometime, it may be easier to prescribe the total amount (grams) of fat and just monitor this along with the cholesterol level. New labeling laws applied to food will help patients and the general public to better understand the concept, however, in depth counseling is essential in facilitating new approaches to eating. In addition, weight reduction and exercise have been shown to reduce triglycerides, lower LDL, raise HDL and lower blood pressure.

A sedentary lifestyle is now considered a key independent risk factor for developing coronary disease. Exercise training has well established benefits such as lower heart rate and blood pressure at rest, increased HDL levels, reduction in anxiety and depression, decreased triglyceride level, and improved glucose tolerance.[13]

Walking appears to be as beneficial as more vigorous exercise when applied with a minimum frequency of 30 to 60 minutes three times a week.[13]

Stress management is an important component of a phase II program. Chronic emotional stress, perceived isolation, lack of social support, hostility, cynicism, and low self-esteem can negatively impact health and healing.[7] Learning to relax and let go, or to altering perceptions about situations and thus the behavior or reaction to a particular event can be life-saving. Sometimes a crises such as hospitalization and surgery can be a turning point for examining lifestyle choices and options. Patients can learn to identify areas in their lives that are difficult and develop strategies and skills for coping successfully. Interventions such as relaxation, imagery, music, meditations and massage can impact healing.[7]

There are many challenges in cardiovascular nursing as we approach the twenty-first century. As the technological development continues, there are monumental pressures to reduce costs, length of hospital stay and improve outcomes. Healthcare providers have the opportunity and the obligation to continue to integrate the concepts of technology, mind, body and spirit into nursing practice, by creating models of health care that facilitate healing and view patients as partners in this process. There is a need to develop innovative programs designed to promote wellness and prevention, to provide expert intervention and follow-up when crisis occurs. As the postoperative interventions are redesigned to assist patients in moving more swiftly through the system, one must also examine the environment and the resources within the system which support healing. As the length of hospital stay decreases, phase II programs will probably need to be redesigned to better meet the needs of a somewhat different patient population. In times of chaos and change, it is important to focus on a clear vision for health care and remain critical and creative thinkers committed to facilitating healing.

REFERENCES

1. Vasquez LT: Cost-containment strategies for centers offering open heart product lines-one conceptual model. Cardiovascular Management, Sept.-Oct., 1993.
2. Cotton P: Fast-track improves CABG outcomes. JAMA 1993;270:2023.
3. Wenger NK, Hellerstein HK: Rehabilitation of the coronary patient. 3rd Edition, Churchill Livingstone, New York, NY, 1992.
4. Guzzetta CE, Dossey BM: Cardiovascular nursing holistic practice. Mosby, St. Louis, MO, 1992.
5. Hanisch P: Informational needs and preferred time to receive information for phase II cardiac rehab patients - what CE instructors need to know. J Cont Educ in Nursing 1993;24:82–89.
6. Burrows SG, Gassert C: Moving right along after open heart surgery. Pritchett and Hull Assoc., Atlanta, GA, 1991.
7. Ornish D: Dr. Dean Ornish's program for reversing heart disease. Ballentine Books, New York, NY 1990.
8. Cardiac Rehabilitation Services. Health Technology Assessment Report. National Center for Health Services Research and Health Care Technology Assessment, Rockville, MD, 1987, No.6.
9. Fletcher GF, Froelicher VF, et al: Exercise standards: a statement for health professionals from the American Heart Association. Circulation 1990;82:2286–2322.
10. Fletcher BJ, Lloyd A, Fletcher GF: Outpatient rehabilitative training in patients with cardiovascular disease - emphasis on training method. Heart and Lung 1988;17(2):199–205.
11. Brown WV: Lipoproteins: what, when, and how often to measure. Heart Disease and Stroke 1992:20–26.
12. Summary of the National Cholesterol Education Program adult treatment panel II report. JAMA 1993;269:3015–3023.
13. Fletcher GF, et al: AHA position statement on exercise. Circulation 1992;86:340–344.

SHIFTING PARADIGMS: PREPARING OURSELVES FOR THE NEXT CENTURY

Jane C. Rothrock, D.N.Sc., R.N.

Delaware County Community College
Media, Pennsylvania

One of the keys to strategic planning is to unlearn basic assumptions so that they can be pulled apart and put back together again in a new configuration. In what is often referred to as the *nanosecond nineties*, change is an irresistible force which requires forgetting some of the old ways to make room for embracing the learning of new ways as we attempt to define and redefine our possible future.

In order to be successful in the next century, those in the business of health care must continually and committedly deal with the future. Such an instinctive exercise in foresight will help them to position where they wish to be, and not where others have placed them. For nursing, the keys to such strategic positioning are anticipation, innovation, and excellence.

Anticipation assists the nursing profession in opportunity identification. Often, the busy times of the nineties see nursing enmeshed in the complexities of day-to-day management, performing more work with less resources, and responding to seemingly diverse, demanding constituencies in the health care arena. Anticipation is different from problem-solving or reacting to the daily situations; it might more properly be thought of as problem-avoidance. To avoid problems, one must strategically explore the future. Since the future is dynamic and not fixed, anticipation requires a deliberate consideration of possible future scenarios that are contemplated with intelligence and imagination. The success may come from divergent, creative thinking followed by focused data, integration, prioritizing the potential, probable, and possible scenarios, gaining useful insights and information in advance of needed action. Information is power, and advanced information enhances and accelerates nursing's path to power in designing its preferred future.

Innovation, another key to strategic positioning, requires nursing to be able to distinguish itself from other health care provider groups. As nursing works to separate the contributions to the institution and to the patient, such contributions must be sought that have applicability to a particular situation. Nursing cannot innovate simply for the sake of innovation; all innovation must have applicability. Finally, excellence becomes the gold standard by which we anticipate and innovate. It is never enough for nursing to be excellent today; nursing must position itself for continual excellence. Excellence is never what it used to be. Nursing has learned that the *status quo* is not the way forward. Instead, nurses must spend less effort in fighting the inevitable and understand more clearly where they are headed. That way, they can use change to their advantage and excel in their ability to master and plan for what may not yet exist.

In order to anticipate, innovate, and excel at change, nurse decision makers require *metanoia*, a mind shift or a completely new way of thinking. In order for that to occur, nurses need to become acquainted with what influences their perceptions and beliefs about the way things are or will be in the future. One way of looking at, and perceiving those influencing factors is to examine our *paradigms*. A paradigm is a set of rules or regulations, that may be implicit or explicit, and establishing the boundaries and perimeters in which to operate. The enormous power of the paradigm lies in the ability to succeed with it. Learning and mastering the rules, there is often reluctance to explore the boundaries or consider changing the rules. This is human nature; paradigms, in and of themselves, are common and functional. However, when the rules strategically blind the ability to anticipate, innovate, and excel, there must be a deliberate attempt to explore them and determine if they still fit the situation and the times.

Paradigm shifts and changes are best undertaken when old paradigms and rules are still in place. It is not advisable to explore paradigms as a reaction to a crisis. Thus, as part of nursing's anticipation of the future, paradigm exploration is a powerful tool. However, the nurse leader who advocates paradigm pliancy, a purposeful exploration and consideration of the future, is often met with resistance. Complacency and comfort with the way things are yields a workforce that does not like the discomfort of rapid, discontinuous change or the spurts and starts of new things that catch them by surprise. In an effort to protect themselves and their investment in the dominant paradigm and set of operant rules, resisters offer the majority of "...Yes, but..." reactions to paradigm exploration. Nonetheless, the nursing leader who deliberately sets the course for paradigm exploration will find that the resistance met is balanced by enormous opportunity. It is this opportunity which beckons and calls to those who wish to remain on the leading edge and participate in designing part of the future.

Health care reform offers nursing a tremendous window of opportunity. The challenge is to contemplate the future scenarios with creative mind sets and not strategic blindness and recognize the potentials and possibilities. It is not difficult to scan the future and see some of the trends on the horizon of change. Health regulation and competition among providers will lead nursing to contemplate new methods for cost containment and collaborative efforts toward regionalization. The anticipated explosion in managed care offers opportunities and concomitant challenges to streamline already tight nursing budgets. As the country explores new financing options for a reformed delivery system, nursing must ensure its negotiating position when national expenditure budgets are addressed. This requires an articulate nursing group that can not only discuss intelligently nursing's agenda for health care reform, but respond to complicated questions regarding financing mechanisms. Anticipated effects of insurance reform will challenge the nursing community to study long- and short-term implications for the institution and the insured in pay or play options. The clear mandate in a reformed system for a balanced equation between quality, cost, and value bodes well for nursing, who has had these as core values for all time. However, collection and dissemination of cost and quality data will challenge the nursing community in terms of its contributions to the equation and its ability to see that its contributions are fairly weighted in terms of patient outcomes. Measurements of what have been elusive outcomes will become a focused goal of qualitative and quantitative nursing research.

As efforts move ahead to document cost and quality, to create innovative delivery systems, to measure patient outcomes, and to offer point-of-care delivery in ambulatory settings, nursing must commit to exploring paradigms and thinking creatively about mechanisms and methods of achieving those goals. Collectively, they must reverse mental locks and prevent strategic blindness from pointing the vision and inquiry in one direction only. Nursing must always seek more than one answer to a question, then weigh the alternatives. They must move away from the mandate to always think logically, to only find the one right answer. Instead, they need to play with ideas, to use soft, imaginative thinking at times, and to allow humor and play to influence their creative attempts at futurist thinking. The worst thing nursing can do at this critical juncture in its history is to believe that it is not creative. Nurses, who have long been educated in process and system thinking, have also developed a strong sense of intuition. It is that ability to take a risk with an idea that feels right, that may not always be based on facts or data which intuitively fits a divergent, creative situation. While statistics are extremely useful in quantitative decision-making, imagination is often as important. Creative thinking combined with knowledge and choices may lead nursing to restructure possible future scenarios. By developing strategies that respond to various scenarios, nursing can rehearse for and play out possible futures. Just as importantly, such strategy development for various creatively imagined alternative futures allows nursing to enhance its ability to reach its preferred outcomes.

Nursing can not risk being too certain of what they *know* based on data; that is the risk of paradigm paralysis, where they become closed to learning new possibilities and perceiving changes. When nursing is open to possibilities,, it is clear that, what worked in the past cannot be depended on to work in the future. The lessons of history, combined with an analysis of recent changes in the health care industry, make it clear that nurses are compelled to undertake a critical evaluation of the probable future environments of their practice. Paradigm exploration allows nursing to approach assumptions about the future deliberatively and systematically, avoiding both, faithful acceptance that the present will continue unchanged, and uncritical acceptance of forecasts of change. Paradigm flexibility will ensure nursing of a future that is not just a matter of chance. As they willingly explore what is possible, probable, and potentially true in their destiny, nurses can make that destiny in part choice. Rather than wait for it to happen, paradigm explorers make their destiny a thing to be achieved.

BIBLIOGRAPHY

Barker J: Future edge: discovering the new paradigms or success. William Morrow Publishers, New York, NY, 1992.
Chinn PL: Looking into the crystal ball: positioning ourselves for the year 2000. Nursing Outlook 1991:39(6):251–256.
Groah L, Howery D: Predictions for perioperative nursing. Nursing 92, 1992:48–49.
Patterson P: What is a paradigm and what makes it shift? OR Manager 1992:18.

CONTRIBUTORS

Susan G. Burrows, R.N., M.N.
Clinical Nurse Specialist
Cardiovascular Surgery
Emory University Hospital
Atlanta, GA

Joan M. Craney, R.N., M.S.N.
Boston College School of Nursing
Boston, MA

Aurel C. Cernaianu, M.D.
Associate Professor Surgery
University of Medicine and
   Dentistry of New Jersey
Robert Wood Johnson Medical
   School
Director of Research Programs
Cooper Hospital/University
   Medical Center
Camden, NJ

Roger S. Damle, M.D.
Assistant Professor of Medicine
Cardiac Electrophysiology
Department of Medicine
Division of Cardiology
University of Colorado Health
   Sciences Center
Denver, CO

Anthony J. DelRossi, M.D.
Professor of Surgery
University of Medicine and
   Dentistry of New Jersey
Robert Wood Johnson Medical
   School
Chairman, Department of Surgery
Head, Division of Cardiothoracic
   Surgery
Cooper Hospital/University
   Medical Center
Camden, NJ

William C. DeVries, M.D.
President, DeVries and Associates
Louisville, KY

Donald B. Doty, M.D.
Clinical Professor of Surgery
University of Utah School of
   Medicine
Chairman, Cardiovascular and
   Thoracic Surgery Division
LDS Hospital
Salt Lake City, UT

Sherry C. Faulkner, C.C.P.
Arkansas Children's Hospital
Little Rock, AR

Jan D. Galla, M.D.
Assistant Professor
Department of Cardiothoracic
   Surgery
The Mount Sinai Medical Center
New York, NY

Timothy J. Gardner, M.D.
William M. Measey Professor of Surgery
Chief, Division of Cardiothoracic Surgery
Hospital of the University of Pennsylvania
Philadelphia, PA

Michele Genoni, M.D.
Clinic for Cardiovascular Surgery
University Hospital
Zurich, Switzerland

Randall B. Griepp, M.D.
Chairman, Department of Cardiothoracic Surgery
Mount Sinai Medical Center
New York, NY

John W. Hammon, Jr., M.D.
Howard Holt Bradshaw Professor of Surgery
Chairman, Department of Cardiothoracic Surgery
Bowman Gray School of Medicine
Wake Forest University
Winston Salem, NC

Alden H. Harken, M.D.
Professor of Surgery
Chairman, Department of Surgery
University of Colorado Health Sciences Center
Denver, CO

Robert B. Karp, M.D.
Professor of Surgery
Chief, Department of Cardiac Surgery
The University of Chicago
Pritzker School of Medicine
Chicago, IL

Patricia A. Kelly, M.D.
Assistant Professor of Medicine
Cardiac Electrophysiology
Department of Medicine
Division of Cardiology
University of Colorado Health Sciences Center
Denver, CO

Mary Ellen Kern, R.N., M.S.N., C.C.R.N.
Critical Care Nurse Specialist
University of Medicine and Dentistry of New Jersey
Robert Wood Johnson Medical School at Camden
Cooper Hospital/University Medical Center
Camden, NJ

Boris Leskosek
Clinic for Cardiovascular Surgery
University Hospital
Zurich, Switzerland

Howard R. Levin, M.D.
Assistant Professor of Medicine
Department of Medicine
Division of Circulatory Physiology
College of Physicians and Surgeons
Columbia University
New York, NY

Debra J. Lynn-McHale, M.S.N., R.N., C.C.R.N.
Clinical Nurse Specialist
Surgical Coronary Care Unit
Thomas Jefferson University Hospital
Philadelphia, PA

David E. Mann, M.D.
Associate Professor of Medicine
Department of Medicine
Division of Cardiology
University of Colorado Health Sciences Center
Denver, CO

Contributors

Patrick M. McCarthy, M.D.
Attending Surgeon
Thoracic and Cardiovascular
  Surgery
Cleveland Clinic Foundation
Cleveland, OH

John L. Ochsner, M.D.
Chief, Thoracic Cardiovascular
  Section
Department of Surgery
Ochsner Clinic
New Orleans, LA

Mahmet C. Oz, M.D.
Assistant Professor of Surgery
Division of Cardiothoracic Surgery
College of Physicians and Surgeons
Columbia University
New York, NY

Julia Ann Purcell, R.N., M.N., C.C.R.N.
Clinical Nurse Specialist
Division of Cardiology
Emory University Hospital
Atlanta, GA

Keith Reemtsma, M.D.
Valentine Mott Professor of Surgery
Chairman, Department of Surgery
College of Physicians and Surgeons
Columbia University
Director of Surgical Services
Presbyterian Hospital
New York, NY

Michael J. Reiter, M.D., Ph.D.
Associate Professor of Medicine
Department of Medicine
Division of Cardiology
Director of Cardiac Arrhythmia
  Services
University of Colorado Health
  Sciences Center
Denver, CO

Eric A. Rose, M.D.
Professor of Surgery
Chief, Division of Cardiothoracic
  Surgery
College of Physicians and Surgeons
Columbia University
New York, NY

Jane C. Rothrock, D.N.Sc., R.N.
Professor of Nursing
Delaware County Community
  College
Media, PA

Jane V. Stewart, M.S.N., R.N., C.C.R.N.
Cardiothoracic Clinical Nurse
Specialist/Consultant
Moorestown, NJ

Marko I. Turina, M.D.
Chief, Department of
  Cardiothoracic Surgery
Professor of Surgery
Clinic for Cardiovascular Surgery
University Hospital
Zurich, Switzerland

Ludwig von Segesser, M.D.
Professor of Surgery
Clinic of Cardiovascular Surgery
University Hospital
Zurich, Switzerland

Branko M. Weiss, M.D.
Institute for Anesthesiology
University Hospital
Zurich, Switzerland

INDEX

Arrhythmogenic, 68, 69
   foci, 144, 145
Abiomed®, 99, 125
Acetylcholine, 161
Activated coagulation time (ACT), 78, 84, 86, 87, 94, 139
Adrenergic agonists, 160
Alprostadil, 159
Amrinone, 160
Aneurysm, 22, 27
   aortic, 2, 58, 83, 85, 111, 166
   dissecting aortic, 167
      left ventricular, 75
   inferior, 75
Angina, 20, 22
   crescendo, 20
Angioplasty, 20, 21, 22, 25, 112, 114
   catheter, 20, 24
   failure, 23, 26
   subclavian flap, 40, 41
Annuloplasty, 9
   commissural, 8
   fusion, 8, 60
   ring, 9
   suture, 7
   tricuspid, 101
Annulus
   aortic, 2, 58
   root, 2
   small aortic, 1
Anterior resection, 9
Anti-tachycardia pacing, 149
Antiarrhythmic, 71, 75, 143, 147
Anticoagulation, 8, 9, 15, 17, 33, 101, 113, 114, 115, 119, 167
Antifibrinolytic, 95, 96
   synthetic, 93
Antihypertensive, 31
Antithrombin III, 86, 87
Aorta
   allograft, 2, 59
   ascending, 28, 30, 32, 35, 60, 61, 100, 110
   arch, 61

Aorta (*cont.*)
   dissection, 29
   coarctation, 39
   descending, 27, 28, 33, 40, 110
      dissections, 35
      thoracic, 83
   distal, 25, 112
   isthmus, 40
   left heart complex, 42
   ventricular components, 1
Aortic
   aneurysms, 83, 113
   arch, 30, 61
   counterpulsation, 109
   cross clamp, 30
   cusps, 7, 59, 60
   dissection, 35
   embolectomy, 72
   homograft, 39
   incompetence, 7
   insufficiency, 18, 31, 34, 111
   junction, 56
   mechanical, 2
   patch angioplasty, 61
   prostheses, 4, 100
   regurgitation, 100
   replacement, 167
   ring, 2, 7
   root, 1, 2, 3, 4, 5, 55, 56, 58, 62
      anatomy, 1
      enlargement, 4
      reconstructions, 31
   sinuses, 7
   stenosis, 17, 100
      surgical treatment, 55
   valve, 1, 2, 7, 31, 32, 59, 61
      annulus, 27
      cusps, 55, 58, 59
      endocarditis, 14
      incompetence, 22, 59, 57, 166
      leaflets, 1
      repair, 18
      replacement, 17, 18, 56, 62, 167
      stenosis, 55, 57, 60, 113

Aortic (*cont.*)
  valvotomy, 62
  valvuloplasty, 57
    degenerative stenosis, 7
Aorto-iliac grafting, 110
Aortography, 28, 29, 31, 166
Aortoplasty, 62
Aortotomy, 4
Aortoventriculoplasty, 4, 59
Aprotinin, 94, 172
Arch, 28, 32
  complete replacement, 30
Arrhythmias, 101
  electroanatomy, 69
  ventricular, 65, 69
Arterial disease
  peripheral, 19
Arterio-venous
  fistula, 53
  hemofiltration, 102
Artery
  axillary, 110
  brachial, 20
  carotid, 40, 109
  circumflex coronary, 8, 20
  femoral, 22, 110
  heterogenous, 46
  iliac, 27
  inferior epigastric, 46, 50
  innominate, 30, 40
  internal mammary, 15, 170
  internal thoracic, 45, 46, 47, 52
  left subclavian, 28
  radial, 51
  right coronary, 20, 50
  right gastroepiploic, 46, 50
  subclavian, 110
  superior epigastric, 48
  wall, 24
  ulnar, 51
Aspirin, 119
Atherectomy, 20
  techniques, 21
Atheromatous plaque, 21
Atrioventricular, 8
Autogenous
  arteries, 46
  skeletal muscle, 122
  veins, 46
Autologous
  blood, 91
  platelet-rich plasma, 91
  pre-donation, 90, 91
  transfusion, 95
Autotransfusion, 85

Barbiturates, 30, 31
Bentall procedure, 30, 31
Beta-blockers, 159, 161

Bilirubin, 103
Biomedicus pump, 30
Bioprostheses, 17
Biventricular, 117, 131
  pulsatile, 116
  replacement prosthesis, 120
  support, 103, 128, 130
    criteria, 126
Blalock-Park technique, 40
Bleeding, 4, 15, 113, 172, 128
Blood
  administration, 103, 158
  component therapy, 89, 173
  conservation, 89, 96
  dyscrasias, 103
  flow, 24
  pressure, 159, 160
  salvage
    postoperative, 92
    red cell, 96
      conservation, 91
  scanning, 20
  substitutes, 89, 92, 95
  transfusion, 89, 90
  whole, 89
Bradyarrhythmia, 65, 149
Bradycardia, 21
Bubble oxygenators, 107
Bypass
  left heart, 77, 79, 81, 82, 85, 107, 109
  veno-venous, 107

Calcification, 15, 21
Calcium channel blockers, 159
  preparation, 161
Cardiac
  arrest, 22
  assist, 106
  cycle, 109
  dysfunction, 135
  enlargement, 17
  index, 100, 125, 127, 157, 159, 160
  ischemia, 19
  output, 3, 4, 107, 111, 119, 157
  pacemaker, 66
  tamponade, 138, 146, 147
  transplantation, 74, 75, 105
Cardiogenic shock, 25, 105, 111, 112, 161
Cardiomyopathy, 101, 102, 111, 116
  hypertrophic, 58
  idiopathic, 119
Cardioplegia, 171
  retrograde, 15, 35, 36
Cardiopulmonary
  arrest, 85
  bypass, 77, 82, 85, 99, 102, 105, 106, 109, 137
    peripheral, 22, 23, 24, 25

Index

Cardiopulmonary (*cont.*)
   resuscitation, 108
Cardiotomy, 85, 113, 116
   cardiac failure, 111
   reservoirs, 85
Cardioversion, 70, 101
Cardioverter, 72
Cardiowest®, 118, 125, 124
Carpentier-Edwards prosthesis, 9, 15
Catheter
   balloon valvotomy, 57
   laser, 21
   right heart, 173
   transatrial, 3
Central venous pressure, 101, 138
Centrifugal
   pump, 36, 83, 116, 124, 130, 131
   support, 124
      cerebral perfusion, 30
Cholesterol, 181
Chorda tendineae, 10
   posterior medial, 9
   rupture, 8
   shortening, 10
   transfer, 10
Circulatory support, 25
Clamp and cut, 35
Claudication, 111
Coagulopathy, 102
Commissure, 2, 5, 10, 55, 59
   fusion, 8, 57, 60
   rudimentary, 57
Compression test, 51
Computed tomography, 28, 31
Concealed entrainment, 146
Conduits, 45
COPD, 159
Coronary, 110
   angiogram, 14
   arterial blockages, 21
   atherosclerosis, 23
   bypass grafting, 7, 10, 13, 15, 16, 17, 18, 19, 20, 22, 25, 26, 46
      artery disease, 3, 16, 19, 75, 101, 105
   collaterals, 68, 69
      button anastomoses, 31
      occlusion, 23
   circulation, 110
   collateral channels, 23
   obstruction, 17
   ostia, 7, 15, 30
   sinus, 8, 67
      cannulation, 24
      perfusion, 24
Counterpulsation, 108, 124
Creatinine, 102
Creatinine phosphokinase, 146
Cryoablation, 145

Cryoprecipate, 137
Cryopreservation, 52
Cusp, 7
   left coronary, 5
   right coronary, 61
Cystic medial necrosis, 165

Deconditioning, 176
Defibrillation, 23
   pacing analyzer, 72
   threshold, 72
Demerol, 172
Desmopressin, 93, 172
Dextran, 129
Dialysis, 102
Diastolic
   augmentation, 109
   pressure, 111
Digoxin, 159, 161
Dilation, 16, 23, 24
Diltiazem hydrochloride, 51, 159
Dipyridamole, 119, 129
Dissection
   type A, 33
   type B, 35, 36
Disseminated intravascular coagulation, 93
Dobutamine, 4, 161
Dopamine, 160
Dopexamine, 160
Doppler
   echocardiography, 3
   ultrasound, 4
Ductus arteriosus, 56
Dynamic
   aortic patch, 109
   cardiomyoplasty, 109, 122
   muscle pump, 109
Dysrhythmias, 166

Echocardiography, 7, 10, 16, 31, 59
ECMO, 83, 114, 124, 135, 138, 139
   neonatal, 136
   support, 124, 136
   veno-venous, 136
   veno-arterial, 138
Ejection fraction, 9
Electrophysiologic studies, 65, 74
Embolization, 21, 23
Endarterectomy, 58, 61
Endocardium, 69
   fibroelastosis, 56
   mapping, 69, 75
   resection, 69, 74
Endothelium-derived relaxing factor, 48
Epinephrine, 159, 160
Epsilon aminocaproic acid, 93, 94, 172
Esmolol, 159

Exercise testing, 179
External
  pulsation pressure, 109
  pumps, 124
  ventricular assistance, 25
Extracorporeal
  lung assist, 83
  mechanical, 100

Flow
  competitive, 16, 50
  probe, 79
  velocity, 48
Fluid replacement, 172
Fluosol-DA, 96
Furosemide, 161

Gastrectomy, 50
Gelatin resorcinol glue, 30
Glucose tolerance, 181
Glutaraldehyde fixation, 52
Goretex
  chorda tendinea, 10, 31
  suture, 9
Graft, 17, 25, 46
  ascending aorta, 167
  Cabrol, 33
  collagen impregnated, 31
  composite, 32
  intraluminal, 36
  replacement, 167
  segmental, 53
  simple patch, 40
Guidewire, 21, 23, 24

HDL, 181
Heart
  mechanical compression, 107
  rate, 157, 159, 160
  right-sided failure, 124
  transplant, 99, 100
Heartmate®, 118, 124
Hemi-arch replacement, 30
Hemodialysis, 102, 130
Hemodilution, 91
Hemodynamic
  collapse, 23
  guidelines, 125
  instability, 19
  performance, 4
  values, 158
Hemoglobin
  concentration, 158
  solutions, 96
Hemolysis, 114, 116
Hemopneumothorax, 72
Hemopumps®, 111, 112, 113, 124
Hemostasis, 137
Hemothorax, 29

Heparin, 77, 84, 86, 94, 117, 120
  coated surfaces, 77, 79, 80, 81, 82, 84, 85, 86, 139
Hepatic
  congestion, 103
  factors, 102, 167
Heparinization, 79, 80, 81, 82, 84, 85, 86
HIS bundle, 67
Histamine, 161
Homologous
  transfusion, 89
  vein, 46, 51
Hyperplasia, 46
Hypertension, 28, 159
Hypoplasia, 40, 41
Hypoplastic left heart syndrome, 42
Hypothermia, 25, 30, 85, 86, 171
Hypothermic circulatory arrest, 30, 32, 33

Infection, 113, 129
Interleaflet triangle, 2, 56, 59
Internal cardioverter defibrillators, 149
Intimal
  disruption, 20
  dissection, 23
  hyperplasia, 47, 48
  tear, 31
Intra-aortic balloon pump (IABP), 22, 23, 103, 105, 108, 110
Ischemia
  cardiomyopathy, 10, 16, 18
  mitral
    incompetence, 10
    regurgitation, 16, 17, 18
  ventricular arrhythmias, 25
Isoproterenol, 160

Konno procedure, 59
Konno-Rastan procedure, 4

Labetalol, 159
Langendorff apparatus, 68
Latissimus dorsi, 122
LDL, 181
Leaflet
  motion, 16
  prolapse, 8, 15
Liquid nitrogen, 68

Magnetic resonance imaging, 28
Marfan syndrome, 29, 30, 32, 166, 167
  thoracic aortic aneurysm, 165
Mechanical ventricular support, 126
Mediastinum, 27
Medtronic-Hall, 4
Membrane oxygenator, 22, 106
Metabolic equivalent of a task (MET), 179
Metaraminol, 161
Milrinone, 160

Mitral incompetence
  congenital, 10
Mixed venous oxygen saturation, 79
Morphine sulfate, 172
Muscle
  papillary, 8, 9, 10, 16
    lengthening, 16
    rupture, 16
Myocardial
  blood flow, 23
  dysfunction, 105
  infarction, 10, 21, 22, 23, 26, 28, 105, 111, 131
  ischemia, 20
  jeopardy, 20
  oxygen consumption, 109, 110
  oxygen demand, 24
  protection, 14, 15, 19
  revascularization, 45, 50, 53, 84
  stunning, 25
Myocardiopathy
  dilated left ventricular, 124
Myxoid degeneration, 17

NADH, 68, 6
Nitrates, 160
Nitroprusside, 160, 161
Non-coronary
  cusp, 5, 61
  sinus, 5
  sinus of Valsalva, 60
Norepinephrine, 160
Normothermia, 23
Novacor®, 124

Operative
  mortality, 41
  risk, 34
Oxygen
  carrying capacity, 158
  consumption, 158
  delivery, 158
  demand, 9
Oxygenators, 84

Pacemaker, 149
Patch, 4
  angioplasty, 41, 61
  aortoplasty, 62
  graft angioplasty, 43
  posterior, 4
Percutaneous transluminal coronary angioplasty (PTCA), 19, 112
Perfluorocarbon solution, 21, 96
Perfluroctyl bromide, 96
Pericardiotomy syndrome, 131
Peritoneal dialysis, 130
Phentolamine, 161
Phenylephrine, 161

Phosphodiesterase inhibitors, 160
Pierce-Donachy Thoratec® VAD, 117
Plasmapheresis, 91
Platelet, 137, 159
  activity, 50
  autologous, 92
  transfusion, 91
Pneumothorax, 72
Polytetrafluroethylene (PTFE), 53
Positive end-expiratory pressure (PEEP), 172
Positive reactive antibody, 100
Pressure
  left atrial, 102, 127, 158
  volume curves, 9
Propranolol, 159
Prostaglandin, 48, 56, 159
Prostheses
  mechanical, 17
Protamine sulphate, 84, 172
Protease inhibitor, 92, 144
Prothrombin time, 103
Pseudo-intima, 118
Pseudomembranous enterocolitis, 109
PT, 117, 129
PTCA, 20, 22, 23
  complications, 20
  failure, 24
  induced coronary artery obstruction, 22
  outcome, 25
  results, 21
  techniques, 21
PTT, 113, 120, 129
Pulmonary
  artery, 110
    catheters, 173
    counterpulsation, 124
    occlusion pressure (PAOP), 106, 158
  diffusion, 102
  emboli, 106
  emoblism, 111
  factors, 102
  hypertension, 102, 159
  resistance, 102
  vascular resistance, 158
  ventilation, 139
Pump
  intravascular, 112
  roller, 77, 79, 82, 106, 109, 138
    left heart bypass, 83
  veno-venous, 139
  oxygenator, 77
  pneumatic, 131

Radiofrequency ablation, 143
Raphe, 55
Re-entry, 144
Recombinant human erythropoeitin, 92, 95
Recurrent subaortic stenosis, 59

Rehabilitation, 176
Renal
  failure, 102, 130
  function, 81
  infarction, 28
Respiratory
  disease, 114
  failure, 137
  rate, 158
Restenosis, 21, 22
Retroperitoneum, 27
Revascularization, 22, 24, 25, 47, 105
Rewarming, 86, 171
Rheumatic disease, 10, 15, 17
Ring
  flexible, 9

Scanning electron microscope, 81
Seldinger technique, 110
Septal myectomy, 58, 59
Septicemia, 111
Sewing rings, 4
Sinus
  tachycardia, 72
  of Valsalva, 2, 55, 60, 61
Skeletal muscle cardiomyoplasty, 99
Sleep cycle, 158
Spasm, 50, 51
Spinal protection, 35
St. Jude, 3, 4, 15
Stents, 23
Steroids, 30, 31
Stroke volume, 119
Subclavian
  prepectoral area, 71
  vein, 72
Subendocardial resection, 73, 145
Subvalvular, 15, 55
Sudden cardiac death, 72, 124
Support
  veno-venous, 137
Supravalvular, 55
  aortic stenosis, 59, 61, 62
SvO$_2$, 173
Synchronized biphasis shock, 72
Syncope, 28
Systemic vascular resistance, 125, 157

Tachyarrhythmia, 65, 69, 74, 149, 159
Tachycardia, 159
Tamponade, 129
Thermo Cardiosystems®, 99
Thoracic
  pain, 28
  spine, 27
Thoratec®, 124, 125
Thromboembolism, 8, 9, 83, 99, 100, 116, 129

Thrombogenicity, 77
Thromboresistant, 85
Thromboses, 9, 27, 33, 147
Thrombotic occlusion, 49
Thrombus, 23
  formation, 101, 113
Thyrocervical branches, 40
Tissue
  oxygenation, 158
  valve, 8
Total artificial heart, 124, 130
Tranexamic acid, 93, 94
Transaminases, 103
Transesophageal echocardiography, 15, 28, 29, 31, 129
Transfusion, 85, 89, 95
Transplantation, 109, 113, 116, 117, 119, 121, 124, 130
Transpulmonary shunt, 137
Transvalvular gradient, 100
Trauma
  craniocerebral, 85
Triangular resection, 7, 9
Trimethaphan, 161
Tubular necrosis, 130
Tunneling procedure, 152

Ultrafiltration, 92
Ultrasonic surgical debridement, 7
Urine output, 81, 125

V-Y flap, 61
Valve, 4, 7, 8, 13, 56, 58
  congenital aortic, 56
  disease, 13
  function, 3
  mitral
    apparatus, 8
    competence, 9
    insufficiency, 100
  native aortic, 8
  orifice, 10
  pathology, 14
  regurgitation, 9, 15, 16, 17
  repair, 8, 10, 15, 16, 167
  replacement, 2, 14, 15
    device, 7
  stenosis, 100
  tensor apparatus, 9
  unicommissural, 55
    stenosis
Valvotomy, 55, 56
Vascular injury, 113
Vasodilator therapy, 50, 172
Vegetations, 15
Vein
  access, 23

Index

Vein (*cont.*)
  bypass grafts, 15, 16
  femoral, 22
  jugular, 109
  saphenous, 16, 45, 49, 53, 170
Ventricular
  activation, 69
  aneurysm, 67, 74, 124
  aortic junction, 7
  apex, 72
  arrhythmias, 17, 65, 101, 111, 113
  assist devices, 99, 102, 105
    complications, 128
    insertion, 103
    placement, 100
    selection, 123
    support, 101
  diastolic pressure, 100
  distention, 22
  dysfunction, 16, 17, 18, 75
  ejection fraction, 84, 159
  end-diastolic pressure, 100, 111, 160
  failure, left-sided, 124, 138
  fibrillation, 72, 73, 101, 124

Ventricular (*cont.*)
  function, 16, 100, 102, 126, 160
  hypertrophy, 3, 16
  outflow tract, 1, 2, 3, 4, 8, 55, 58, 59
  pacing, 65, 66, 72
  performance, 112, 160
  pressures, 109, 158
  right, 15, 117, 125
  septal defect, 41
  septum, 59, 61
  shortening, 9
  stroke volume, 138
  support, 111, 114, 117, 120, 130
  tachycardia, 63, 67, 68, 69, 71, 73, 74, 75, 143, 144
  wall stress, 110
Ventriculoartic junction, 1
Ventriculography, 15
Verapamil, 159
VT foci
  identification, 146

Warfarin, 17, 117, 120, 129